DEADLY PERILS

COASTAL SHIPPING AND SHIPWRECK AROUND PEMBROKESHIRE AND THE ISLANDS

"The Bishop and these his Clerkes preache deadly doctrine to their winter audience."
George Owen

PETER B. S. DAVIES

MERRIVALE

All rights reserved. No part of this publication may be reproduced, stored in a retrieval system or transmitted in any form or by any means electronic, photocopying, recording or otherwise, without the prior permission of the author.

Extract from Register of ships loading coal and culm at Nolton Haven for the period 8th - 11th May, 1849; five of the ships named were later lost off the Pembrokeshire Coast, while *Heart of Oak* was wrecked in 1887 at Llangrannog.

Copyright; Peter B. S. Davies 1999

First Edition 1992 (ISBN 0 9515207 2 5)
Second (Revised & Enlarged) Edition 1999

ISBN 0 9515207 8 4

Acknowledgements

I am deeply grateful to the staffs of the County Record Offices at Haverfordwest, Aberystwyth and Carmarthen for their help and for enabling me to consult the Shipping Registers and the Log Books and Crew Lists for the West Wales ports; also the Marine Safety Agency at Llanishen, Cardiff, who hold the most recent Registers. My thanks are also due to the staffs of the National Library of Wales, Aberystwyth; Haverfordwest Reference Library; Carmarthen Reference Library; St. David's Cathedral Library; who (together with Haverfordwest Record Office) provided copies of early newspapers and a variety of other documents.

Among individuals, Lewis Lloyd supplied information on Aberdyfi and Barmouth vessels; Les Owen gave details from his researches into early Shipping Registers held at the Public Record Office, Kew; Benjamin Harries extracted information on the careers of seamen from records at the National Maritime Museum, Greenwich; while George Harries gave much help and advice, particularly with regard to trade with Bristol. To all I am much indebted.

For permission to reproduce photographs I am grateful to St. David's Cathedral Library (5), Haverfordwest Reference Library (7) and the National Library of Wales (11). Facsimiles of documents are by permission of Haverfordwest Record Office.

Finally I am particularly indebted to David Chant (formerly coxswain of the St. David's Lifeboat) for the cover photograph of the lifeboat *Joseph Soar* rounding the southern end of Ramsey Island. Taken from his motor fishing vessel, it graphically illustrates the hazards which the crews of the old time sailing vessels had to face.

Published by Merrivale, St. David's
Printed by C.I.T., Haverfordwest

Cover: St. David's Lifeboat *Joseph Soar* rounding Ynys Beri at southern end of Ramsey Island; photograph by David Chant

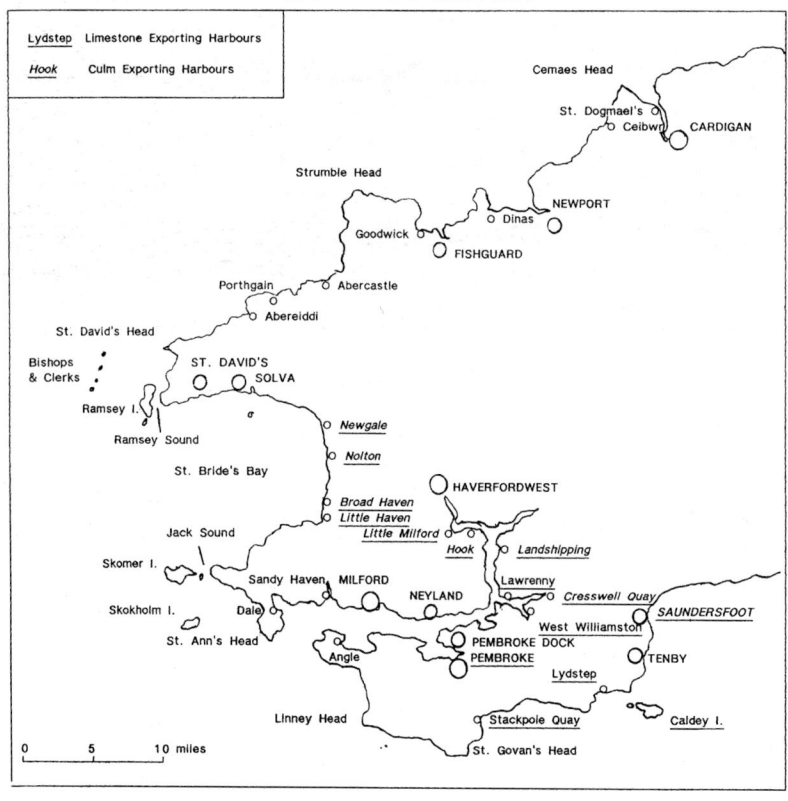

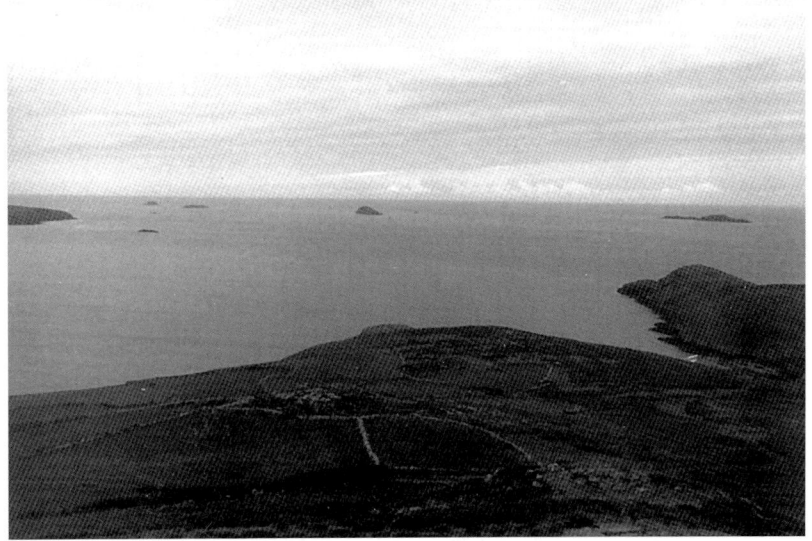

1. *Octopitarum Promontorium* from the slopes of Carnllidi; North Bishop behind St. David's Head, Carreg Rhosson, Daufraich and South Bishop, with Ramsey Island on left.

Contents

	The Eight Perils	7
I	Hard Facts of Rocks	10
II	The Hidden Menace	15
III	The Great Gale	20
IV	Collision Course	25
V	The Final Straw	29
VI	Crossing the Bar	33
VII	No Hiding Place	38
VIII	Death of a Veteran	42
	List of Shipwrecks	46
	Bibliography	56

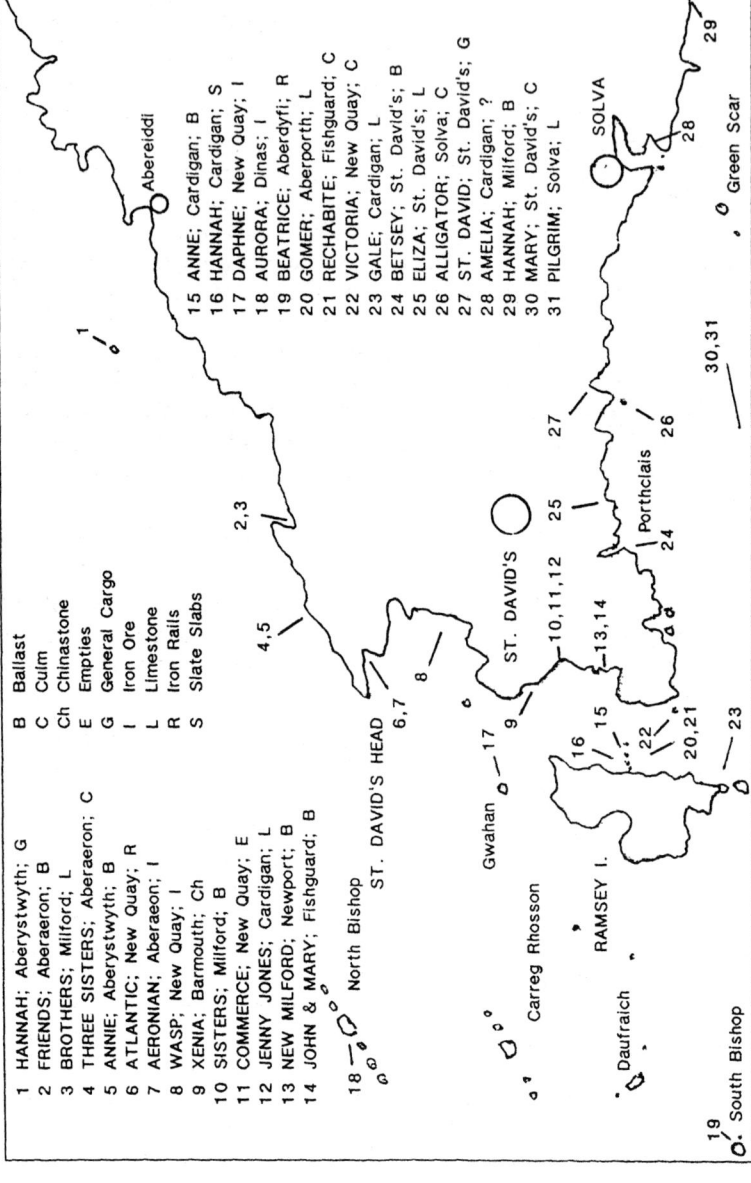

The Eight Perils

The second century Alexandrian geographer Ptolemy gave the name *Octopitarum Promontorium* (Headland of Eight Perils) to this remote and secret place. Today, more prosaically, it is known as Penmaen Dewi or St. David's Head. The origins of the name are long forgotten, but tradition associates the perils with the Bishops and Clerks, the miniature archipelago that lies beyond Ramsey.

On a clear summer's evening the islands seem to float on the horizon, a granite flotilla; North Bishop, Carreg Rhosson, Daufraich and South Bishop. Four small islands, none more than a few acres in extent, each with its attendant clerks - lonely, mysterious. But during a winter storm, when the mighty Atlantic waves foam around the islands and cascade over the lesser rocks and reefs, it becomes a place of menace.

Apart from the (now automatic) lighthouse on South Bishop, none of the islands has ever been inhabited, though, in the past, the main islands were used for grazing a few sheep during the summer months. Otherwise they produced gulls' eggs, some of which were eaten locally, while others were sent to Bristol for use in the fining of wine. Today the islands belong to the seabirds and the seals.

The islands and their surrounding waters have always been feared by seamen. In the words of the Elizabethan historian, George Owen:

> "These rocks are accounted sore daunger to those that seeke Milford coming from the south-west seas .... The Bishop and these his Clerkes preache deadly doctrine to their winter audience, such poor seafaring men as are forcyd thither by tempest."

Not until 1839 was the lighthouse erected on the South Bishop to warn mariners of the dangers, and it was 1869 before the first St. David's lifeboat arrived.

In 1850, after acting for several years as a deputy agent, Samuel Williams, a local merchant, was appointed Lloyd's Agent for St. David's, responsible for the coast from Abereiddi to Newgale. Nearly two decades later he drew up a list of the ships he could recall being wrecked in that area. The surviving draft is incomplete and contains a few errors, nevertheless it provides a fascinating insight to the shipping of those days.

Nearly seventy ships are listed, together with, in most cases, their home port, the cargo they carried, and the site of the wreck. About half were sea-going ships from Liverpool and other distant ports, but over thirty belonged to the little harbours along the coast between Milford and Barmouth. In spite of the fact that early shipping registers of the West Wales ports are incomplete, while vessels of under 15 tons were not recorded on the register, most of these can be positively identified.

A few were larger vessels not engaged in local trading. One of these was the two-masted schooner *Aeronian* of Aberaeron, carrying iron ore, which was wrecked at Porth Melgan on 21st October, 1856; at 44 tons she was smaller than some of the single-masted sloops - the 'Dirty British Coasters' of their day. Only slightly larger was the 50 ton schooner *Feronia* of Llanelli, the only Carmarthenshire-owned vessel on the list. It was on New Year's Day, 1852, that she foundered in St. Bride's Bay; she also was laden with iron ore.

There was nothing romantic about the sloops or their trade. Most were less than forty feet in length and broad in the beam, with flat bottoms to enable them to sit upright on the beaches; they carried between twenty and fifty tons of cargo. Their voyages took them not to some foreign shore in search of treasure but usually to Milford Haven and South Pembrokeshire to load culm and limestone.

Three Sisters was homeward bound to Aberaeron when she was wrecked in 1829. According to the cathedral burial register her master was John Williams, aged 22, "whose vessel with two others was stranded near St. David's Head on Friday 5th July; every soul on board the three perished except one was thrown on the cliff." *Victoria* was making for New Quay when, at about 11 a.m. on Sunday, 9th February, 1845, she struck the Shoe Rock at the southern end of Ramsey Sound; her crew escaped by boat. Both sloops were loaded with culm. Sailing home with cargoes of limestone were *Jenny Jones* of Cardigan, wrecked near Porth Stinan, and *Gomer* of Aberporth which foundered in Ramsey Sound.

Some had come from further afield, perhaps from Bristol. *Hannah* of Aberystwyth was returning with general cargo when she struck one of the rocks off Abereiddi. *Commerce* was carrying empty barrels home to New Quay when she was wrecked in Ramsey Sound on Tuesday, 6th August, 1844. Nearby the same gale drove ashore the 45 ton sloop *Xenia* of Barmouth; she too became a total loss, though most of her cargo of chinastone (not all the sloops traded locally) was transferred to small craft and landed at Porthclais. Fortunately the crews of both sloops were saved.

Ships bound for Milford and the Bristol Channel were usually in ballast. Among these were *New Milford* of Newport and *John & Mary* of Fishguard, both of which were wrecked in Ramsey Sound. On 27th August, 1829, the 18 years old Cork-built smack *Sisters* was also wrecked in Ramsey Sound; she had been purchased from her former owners by Major Samuel Harries of Trevaccoon in Llanrhian parish only six weeks earlier. The year 1829 was a particularly unlucky one for the Major, his previous sloop, the two years old *Lady Melville*, having been "lost at sea"; a not uncommon fate for the coastal traders. But *Hannah* of Cardigan was carrying slate slabs when she sank north of the Bitches at the Waterings.

Two thirds of the losses among the local craft took place near St. David's Head or in Ramsey Sound. Other vessels were lost in St. Bride's Bay. *Pilgrim* of Solva with limestone and *Mary* of St. David's with culm both foundered in the bay; *Hannah* of Milford, in ballast, was wrecked near Porth Mynawyd, while *Betsey* of St. David's, also in ballast, was lost near the entrance to Porthclais Harbour.

Of all the local ships lost in the area, two only - *Aurora* of Dinas (probably carrying iron ore) wrecked on North Bishop, and the 84 ton schooner *Beatrice* of Aberdyfi (loaded with iron rails) which struck South Bishop - went ashore on the Bishops and Clerks themselves. Neither was engaged in local trade. *Beatrice*, under her master Josiah James, was on passage from Cardiff to Liverpool when, on the evening of 22nd August, 1859, in dense fog, the tides carried her onto the rocks. The seas remained calm, and nearly 48 hours later due largely to the efforts of Captain John Rees, the local Lloyd's Agent, she was refloated on the rising tide and brought into Solva. *Beatrice* suffered relatively little damage; few if any other vessels escaped after being stranded on the Bishops and Clerks.

Other lists of wrecks confirm that few sloops fell victim to the 'Deadly Doctrine'. It was the larger sailing vessels and steamships trading to and from the Irish Sea which came to grief on these rugged offshore islands.

The local sailors heeded the warnings and avoided the Bishops and Clerks, But they could not avoid Ramsey Sound and the waters around St. David's Head. There were other headlands: Dinas, Strumble, St. Ann's, Linney, and many more; and there was Jack Sound. There were the ever-changing tides, the unexpected storms and the all-enveloping fogs. Then, at the end of an arduous voyage, the crew, cold and exhausted, had to bring the vessel safely through the narrow and hazardous entrance to the harbour.

Few of the local sloops fell prey to the 'Eight Perils' themselves. But there were other dangers equally great lying in wait all around the Pembrokeshire coast.

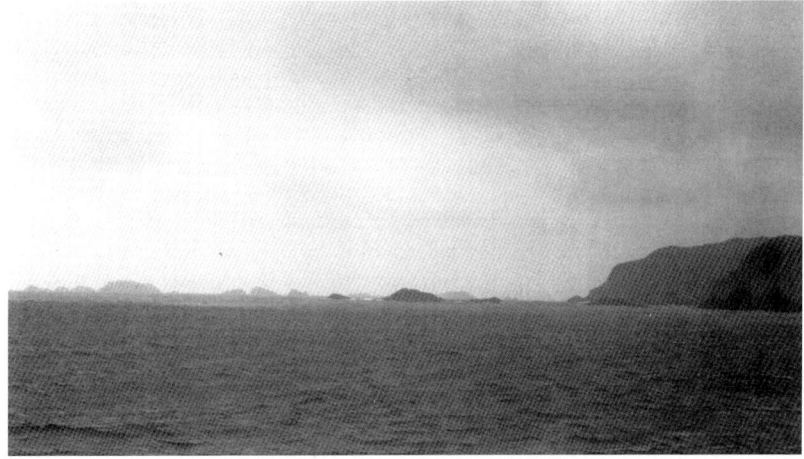

2. Panorama of Perils from St. Bride's Bay; Ynys Beri and west side of Ramsey Island (extreme right); Meini Duon (centre foreground) with North Bishop on horizon; Carreg Rhosson and attendant Clerks (left).

I; Hard Facts of Rocks

In the late twentieth century, Milford Haven is synonymous with the oil industry; giant tankers bring cargoes of a hundred thousand tons and more of crude oil to its refineries from all corners of the world. In the two previous centuries, the Haven meant culm and limestone. The ships were very different, mostly single-masted sloops carrying less than fifty tons of cargo; but, in their time, they were even more significant to the local economy than are the tankers of today.

They came from all the little creeks and harbours of West Wales; and they came in their hundreds. To reach Milford they had to sail around the rock-girt Pembrokeshire coast with its succession of promontories stretching far out to sea. Each, with its underwater reefs and its treacherous currents, presented a challenge to the sailor. Each was different, and each could be deadly to the mariner who was unwary or even unlucky.

On Monday, 18th February, 1861, the 20 ton smack *Elizabeth & Mary*, built seven years earlier at Pembroke Dock, set out from Milford with a cargo of culm bound for her home port of Newport. By evening a strong south-easterly wind was blowing, and Captain Jenkins decided to shelter overnight in Fishguard Bay. About 11 p.m., as he was approaching the bay, a sudden squall carried away the smack's foresail. With the ship partly disabled, the master elected to run for shelter in Carreg Onnen Roadstead, in the lee of Strumble Head. Next morning around 6 a.m., the wind suddenly veered south-west and increased yet further. No longer protected by the bulk of the headland, the ship, trapped within the confines of the little bay, was at the mercy of wind and wave. There was no sandy beach, as at Goodwick, where the ship could as a last resort be run ashore, and all depended on the anchor holding. But, within a short time, the fury of the storm caused the chain to part, and the helpless sloop was driven ashore on the jagged rocks of Carreg Onnen Island.

As the ship struck the rocks and began to break up, the master and mate managed to struggle through the raging surf to the island, but the boy, who was the third member of the crew, was swept to his death. Only at first light was the wreck discovered by two labourers from the nearby farm of Llanwnwr. They summoned assistance, but it seemed that little could be done immediately to aid the two survivors, one of whom could be seen clinging desperately to an outlying rock over which the waves swept incessantly.

Carreg Onnen lies immediately west of Ynys Meicel on which the lighthouse was later erected. There seemed to be no possibility of reaching the survivors from the shore, and Mrs. Mortimer of Llanwnwr despatched a messenger to Fishguard to summon the lifeboat. Obviously a considerable time must elapse before the lifeboat could reach the scene of the disaster. Meanwhile the two seamen were in constant danger of being swept from their precarious positions.

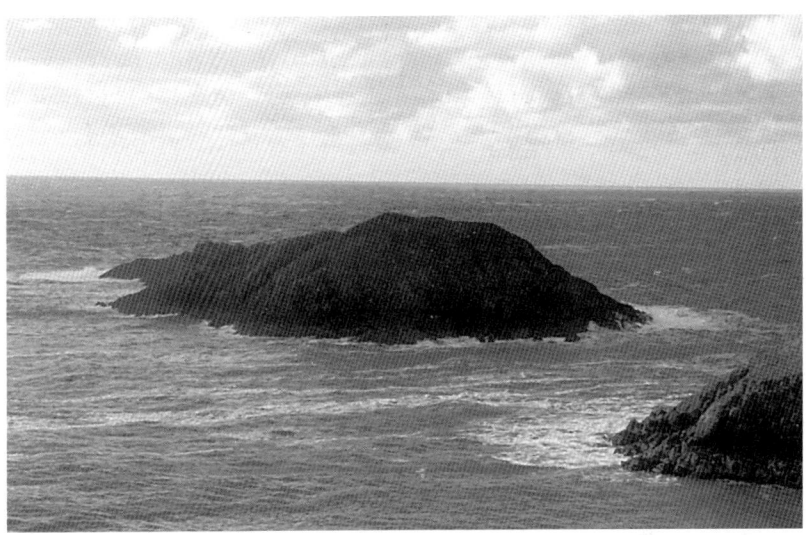

3. Carreg Onnen, near Strumble Head, scene of the wreck of the smack *Elizabeth & Mary*.

By this time a considerable crowd had gathered on the clifftop to watch the unfolding drama. David Beddoe, a sailor from Fishguard, realised that the survivors would almost certainly perish before the lifeboat arrived and volunteered to attempt to swim to the island with a rope. After a Herculean effort he reached the island, where he was shortly afterwards joined by Albert Furlong of the Great Western Hotel, Main Street, Fishguard. Together they managed to throw a rope to the mate and succeeded in hauling him to the shore. They then brought the master to safety before the lifeboat arrived.

The story is told in some detail in the *Haverfordwest and Milford Haven Telegraph* of 20th February. Six weeks later the paper announced that the Royal National Lifeboat Institution had awarded silver medals to the two heroic rescuers. They were also presented with two guineas by John Phillips Esq.. Although the lifeboat, after a long and arduous voyage, arrived too late to take part in the rescue, the crew members were awarded £6 by the Institution for their efforts.

The master and mate were extremely fortunate to escape with their lives. To many of the wrecks on this rocky and lonely coast there were no witnesses; even where there were, they were often powerless to help. Apart from Fishguard, where a lifeboat station was founded in 1822 (it was taken over by the Royal National Lifeboat Institution in 1855) it was only in the second half of the nineteenth century that the local lifeboat stations were established. By then the coastal trade was well past its peak. Although these early lifeboats performed many gallant rescues, their slow speed and limited range meant they had little hope of reaching in time any ship wrecked on one of the remote headlands or islands.

The unfortunate *Elizabeth & Mary* was not the only Newport coaster to come to grief on Strumble Head. Ten years later, on 3rd April 1871, the 21 ton, Hull-built, *Exley* went aground nearby and became a total loss. Her master, 58 years old John Jones, and mate, David Llewellyn aged 60, both perished. Re-registered at Cardigan in 1861, her time was mostly spent bringing culm and limestone to Newport. During the first half of 1866 she made three voyages from Pembrey with coal and six (cargo unspecified) from Milford for her owner Eliza Berriman. In the following six months, she carried a further four cargoes of limestone and five of culm from Milford to Newport.

Elizabeth Berriman had also been the sole owner of the 18 ton smack *Richard & Mary*. The Cardigan Register contains the brief entry: "lost 1854." Similar entries occur frequently in the various registers; often they imply that the ship set out on a voyage but never reached its destination, no trace of vessel or crew being found. A few disappearances are briefly reported in local papers; *Wombwell*, of and from Cardigan, in a severe gale in 1839 while on a voyage to Milford; *Ant* of Pembroke Dock, whose master was unfamiliar with the passage, in 1865 while carrying culm from Sprinkle Pill to St. David's. However the *Haverfordwest and Milford Haven Telegraph*, dated 25th October, records that *Richard & Mary* had parted her cables in Fishguard Bay and had gone ashore at Betws Point. A fortnight later she was still aground, eventually becoming a total wreck.

On 6th August, 1860, the 33 ton sloop *Comet*, under her master David Thomas, was making for her home port of Aberystwyth from Newport (Gwent) with a cargo of coal. While attempting to round Strumble Head in an increasingly severe north-east gale she 'parted her shrouds' - the ropes supporting the mast. Drifting helplessly, she was eventually driven ashore beneath the near-perpendicular cliffs at Aberfelin, near Trefin.

The small boat was launched, but was immediately swept from their grasp, leaving the two men and a boy stranded on the sloop which was already breaking up. The local coastguards had seen the *Comet* strike and made their way to the scene where, after bravely climbing down the cliff, they succeeded in catching and making fast a hawser thrown by the shipwrecked mariners.

The mate clambered over this to the shore with comparative ease. He was followed by the boy, who reached halfway before losing his grip and falling shrieking into the water. Without pausing for thought James Salter, one of the coastguards, plunged in after him; after a heroic struggle in the boiling seas the coastguard landed the boy on a nearby strip of sand. The master, who had been injured during the storm, still clung to the rapidly disintegrating *Comet*. The rescuers could do little to help. Painfully, inch by inch, he had to drag himself along the rope to safety. It was, as the *Pembrokeshire Herald* of 17th August reported, 'a miraculous escape.'

On 6th June, 1857, it was a dense fog which led to the Fishguard smack *Lilly*, in ballast for Lydstep, running aground near Linney Head; she was expected to become a total loss. Built at Bideford in 1798 she had only recently been purchased by her master Captain Rees; unlike many of her kind she was fully insured. The damage was not as bad as first thought, and, some three weeks later, after strenuous efforts of over twenty labourers who dug a channel to the sea, the smack was refloated and towed to Milford, the first vessel to be salvaged from the south end of Freshwater West.

During the great gale of October, 1859, *Lilly* was one of two vessels driven against Fishguard Bridge; again, though damaged, she escaped. However, nine years later her luck finally ran out when, on 12th September, 1868, *Lilly* was lost near Strumble Head.

It was not only the great headlands that claimed their victims, and bad weather was not always to be blamed for the loss. On 14th September, 1858, the smack *Alligator* of Solva was making her way homewards in ballast from Fishguard. As she was working her way up the coast of St. Bride's Bay, she failed to go about and struck the rocky islet of Penpleidiau where she became a total wreck. The crew scrambled onto the rock, from which they were rescued by a boat from nearby Porthclais.

Like the other vessels, *Alligator* was mainly engaged in carrying culm and limestone from Milford, though she did on occasion take corn to Bristol. In this context 'Milford' did not refer to the town itself, but to the Haven, and in particular its upper reaches. In the accounts of voyages given in the 'Log Books and Crew Agreements', the actual point of loading is rarely mentioned. Enormous quantities of limestone were exported annually to feed the limekilns which were to be found all around the coast. By far the most important source of the limestone was West Williamston on the Carew River. There were other important quarries beside the river below Pembroke, as well as much smaller ones south of Haverfordwest.

The principal coal mining district on Milford Haven was around Hook. Towards the end of the eighteenth century, several quays were constructed along the Cleddau to facilitate the loading of the ships; most of these were eventually served with tramways and inclines leading from the mines. Among the more important quays were those at Little Milford, Hook and Lower Hook. Quays were also established at Landshipping to serve the mines on the eastern side of the river and at Cresswell on one of the lesser branches of the Haven.

Culm was also obtained from the St. Bride's Bay Coalfield, most being exported from Nolton. However the mines were small, and produced powdery anthracite, best suited for use as fuel in limekilns. There were few facilities on the west-facing loading beaches, which could only be used during the summer months. Not surprisingly, the coalfield was never properly developed.

Far more important was Saundersfoot on Carmarthen Bay. Here, too, the culm was originally loaded from open beaches such as Wiseman's Bridge and Amroth, but in 1829 a proper harbour was constructed at Saundersfoot. An extensive four foot gauge railway system (later steam operated) was developed, linking each of the main collieries in the Kilgetty and Begelly areas with its own wharf at the harbour.

Ships from the north bound for Saundersfoot had to sail along the south coast of the county to reach their destination. However, the precipitous limestone cliffs of the Castlemartin peninsula claimed comparatively few victims among the local coasters. Some sloops from Milford and beyond did come this way to fetch high grade anthracite from Saundersfoot and house coal from Glamorganshire; others were 'Bristol Traders'. But they were relatively few. As well as coal at Saundersfoot, there was limestone near Tenby and at Lydstep and on Caldey Island from which it was exported. Ships from Tenby and Carmarthen had no need to visit the Haven for these vital commodities.

One of the craft lost here was the *Waft* of Tenby. A 24 ton sloop, built at Llanddewi Aberarth in 1813, she was originally registered at Cardigan. In 1822 she was purchased by John Evans, mariner, of St. David's and re-registered at Milford. Then, in 1829, she was sold to two Tenby mariners; David Rees (43 shares) and Thomas Lloyd (21 shares); the latter became master of the sloop. The south coast of the county is an inhospitable shore, lacking in harbours, and with no shelter from the ceaseless Atlantic swell. The crumbling limestone crags are as deadly as the granite masses of the north. The near vertical cliffs afford little prospect of survival to the shipwrecked mariner. In the end they claimed *Waft* among their victims. Her entry in the Milford Register ends: "Vessel and register lost at St. Govan's Head in 1836." Of the fate of her crew there is no mention.

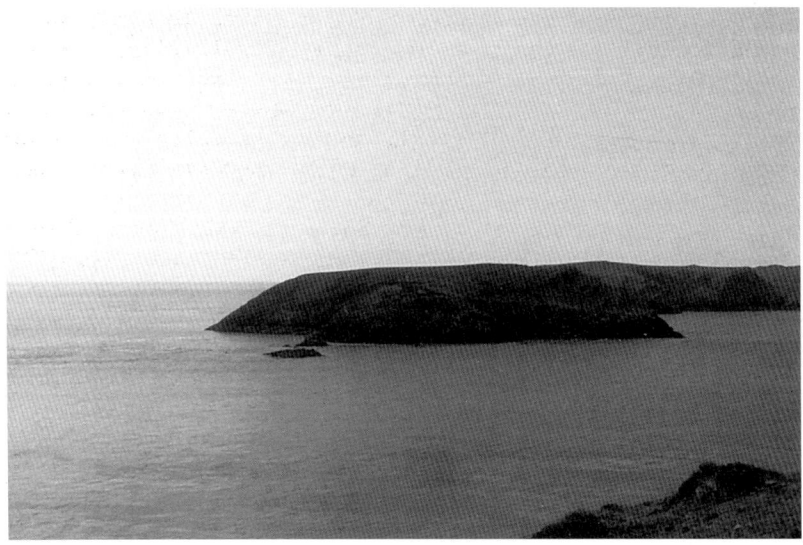

4. Jack Sound from Wooltack Point, looking towards the Crabstones, Midland Island and Skomer.

II; The Hidden Menace

From time immemorial the rock-strewn waters of the southern approaches to the Irish Sea have been feared by seafarers. Best known of the offshore reefs are the Smalls, on which a remarkable lighthouse was erected in 1776 to warn sailors of their lurking presence. Even so, they (and their neighbours the Hats and the Barrels) continued to claim their unsuspecting prey as, nearer to shore, did the Bishops and Clerks themselves.

Apart from the sloops trading with Ireland the local coastal shipping did not normally venture into these waters. Those which were lost mostly vanished without trace. One such was the *Fanny & Betsey* of Pembroke, owned by Sir John Owen, which left Wicklow in company with another of his ships in January 1832, but never arrived in the Haven.

More fortunate were the crew of the sloop *Diligence* of Aberdyfi. The *Carmarthen Journal* records how, on 4th January, 1843, while in the vicinity of Grassholm, she was dismasted during a severe gale. With the vessel sinking, and no possibility of outside help, the crew took to the small boat. After rowing a dozen or so miles in appalling conditions, the survivors succeeded in reaching the safety of Porthclais Harbour.

To avoid the outer islands, the bulk of the coastal shipping kept close inshore, sailing inside the larger islands of Ramsey, Skomer and Skokholm. This, too, had its dangers, as the ships had to navigate through the narrow passages of Ramsey Sound and Jack Sound with their underwater rocks and the powerful unseen currents, which lured ships, siren-like, towards them.

Ramsey Sound runs roughly north - south between the island and the mainland; nearly two miles in length, it has a depth of over sixty feet. For most of its length it is more than half a mile wide, except near its southern end. Here, opposite the headland of Penmaenmelyn with its ruined copper mine, the saw-toothed reef of the Bitches stretches almost halfway across the sound. The other principal hazard is the usually submerged rock the Horse (Ceffyl) opposite Porth Stinan.

About eight miles to the south, Jack Sound separates Midland Island, a smaller island east of Skomer, from the mainland at Wooltack Point. The sound is almost half a mile wide and is comparatively short, but it contains a number of rocks and reefs which make it as deadly as its northern neighbour. Near Wooltack Point is Tusker Rock, off Midland lie the Crabstones, while directly opposite, near Anvil Point, visible only at low water is the Cable. To the south of the narrows are the Black Stones on the west of the channel, with the Bench on its eastern side.

Between Caldey Island and the mainland is the relatively innocuous Caldey Sound, while the islands of Skomer and Skokholm are separated by Broad Sound. The latter, though free of rocks, is much feared because of the nearby Wild Goose Race - a mass of tumbled waters where two tidal currents meet. Fortunately it was off the course of most of the coastal traders.

Elsewhere around the coast are isolated underwater hazards; Llechau, off Abereiddi; Half Tide Rock, off Porthclais; Crow Rock, near Linney; rocks which show themselves only at low tide.

In 1830 there were, according to Pigot, four 'Bristol Traders' based in Haverfordwest which between them kept up a fairly regular weekly service with that city throughout the year. One of the longest serving of these was the *Liberty*, at 69 tons unusually large for a sloop. Her fourteen owners included her master Henry Williams and two Bristol merchants; the remainder were mainly from Haverfordwest itself.

Liberty, laden with a cargo including corn and butter, set sail from Milford about 10 a.m. on 30th April, 1831; there was a light breeze from the north and the sea was calm. After rounding Linney Head, while attempting to pass inside the Crow Rock, she struck the outlying reef known as the Toes. The sloop fell over into deep water and began to sink, giving the crew of four and nine passengers barely time to launch the small boat. Fortunately the sea remained calm and all were picked up by the *Earl of Kingston*, another Bristol Trader, and landed at Milford at 11 p.m. that night. Only the previous month the paddle-steamer *Frolic* had been lost at Nash Sands while on the same route, with the loss of all seventy odd souls aboard.

Whenever possible, ships would use the tidal flow to carry them through the sounds. David Evans of Porthmawr, who kept a diary during the 1840s, wrote that it was not unusual to see sixty or even eighty small craft passing

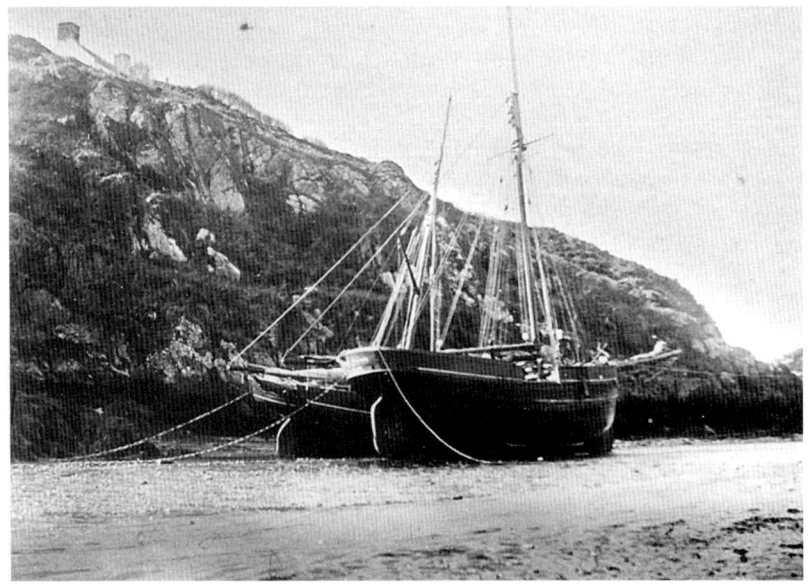

5. Coastal traders at Porthclais, c. 1890; the nearer vessel is the smack *Edith Williams* of St. David's, the other is possibly the cutter *Martha Jane*.

through Ramsey Sound on a single tide. Most belonged to ports further north, and, not surprisingly, some came to grief during the passage.

The *Haverfordwest and Milford Haven Telegraph* of 13th April, 1859, contains a letter from Captain Evans of the smack *Wasp* of New Quay, which had run on a rock in Ramsey Sound on 1st April. In it he expresses, on behalf of the crew, thanks "to those who so kindly (and in peril of their lives) rendered assistance at the time of their misfortune." He is especially grateful to Mr. Bowen of Trelethin for providing them with hospitality.

Even seamen with a lifetime's experience of these waters could meet with disaster in Ramsey Sound. On 19th March, 1894, the cutter *Martha Jane* (master Thomas Tudor, Lower Moor, St. David's) owned by William Williams, Grove Hotel, St. David's, was wrecked on the Bitches; her crew, and most of her cargo of (artificial) manure, were saved. In the previous year she had carried a variety of cargoes to Porthclais; culm from Nolton and Hook, limestone from Milford, timber and manure from Pembroke Dock. She had taken culm from Nolton to Porthgain, and sailed from there with stone for Milford and bricks for Porthclais. And from Porthclais there had been one cargo of grain for Laugharne.

Built at Cosheston in 1872, *Martha Jane* had originally been owned by Thomas Jones of Front Street, Pembroke Dock. Throughout 1874 and the first half of 1876 she had operated within the Haven. During the second half of 1876 she had sailed to Newport (Gwent), Swansea, Saundersfoot and Little Haven, probably to load coal. Inside the Haven she had visited Pembroke, Milford and Dale as well as Pembroke Dock.

Ships passing through Jack Sound had to follow a dog-leg course to avoid the rocks, and the dangerous currents in these confined waters led to many vessels being lost. A singularly unfortunate owner was Michael James, farmer and merchant, of Solva. On 16th October, 1837, his 28 ton, Solva-built sloop *Jane* was wrecked in Jack Sound. Barely eighteen months later, on 11th May, 1839, her replacement the 17 ton smack *Industrious* was lost nearby, together with her master John Phillips and crew. Her successor the sloop *Anne* was more fortunate, surviving (under several owners) until 1885 when she was broken up.

A curious tale concerns the *Sea Horse* which was wrecked in Jack Sound on 21st November, 1831, while on passage to Abereiddi with culm. Ten months later a body was washed up at Abereiddi and interred in nearby Llanrhian churchyard. It was subsequently identified (according to one version of the story, by stockings of unusual pattern which his wife had knitted) as that of Richard Propert of Pembroke Dock, master of the sloop.

The *Dewsland and Kemes Guardian* of Saturday, 14th August, 1880, describes the loss of the 21 ton New Quay smack *Ann Davies* which had taken place five days previously. Homeward bound, while attempting the passage through Jack Sound, her master Henry Davies had misjudged the strength of the currents, and the vessel had been carried by the tide against the cliffs of Midland Island. So severe had been the impact that she had sunk almost immediately. Fortunately the master and his only companion John Jones (described as 'mate and cook' in the crew list) had managed to escape.

The smack had been built at Traethgwyn in 1863 and registered at Aberystwyth in that year, when her sole owner was Evan Timothy, merchant, of New Quay. In the register the site of her loss is given as, "at entrance of St. Bride's Bay." During her final year *Ann Davies* had completed two voyages from Swansea and one each from Porthcawl, Llanelli and Pembrey, presumably with coal. There was one voyage from Lydstep with limestone and five from Milford. Twice her destination was New Quay and once Aberaeron; the other voyages were to Llangrannog. On her fateful twelfth voyage she was again bound from Milford to Llangrannog.

Another vessel lost in Jack Sound was *Mary*, a 45 ton sloop which had been built at Lawrenny in 1802. For much of her career she was owned by Stephen Hurlow, farmer, of Lower Castleton in Monkton parish. Her home port at this time would have been the ancient town of Pembroke.

On 24th August, 1853, *Mary* was registered again at Milford on account of change of ownership. Her new owner was John Rowe, described in 1858 as a coal merchant of Water Street, Pembroke Dock; one of a new class of merchants and shipowners then appearing in the towns of the county. However, his ownership of *Mary* was not to survive the year.

The transfer of the ship from Pembroke to nearby Pembroke Dock mirrored the changes that were taking place on the Haven. For centuries, the trade had been dominated by the Norman boroughs of Pembroke and Haverfordwest. But, during the early nineteenth century, three new towns were to spring up on the shores of the waterway; Milford, originally a whaling settlement; Pembroke Dock, a naval dockyard; and Neyland, a ferry port for Ireland.

The pre-eminence of Pembroke and Haverfordwest dated from Norman times, when their castles had been established overlooking the lowest crossing points - and heads of navigation - of two of its branches. Their dominance, along with Tenby, of Pembrokeshire's trade continued into the Elizabethan era, when the Port of Milford, with its chief Custom House on the quay at Pembroke, became Head Port for the coast between Worm's Head and Barmouth.

The accounts of the voyages of Abel Hicks - who traded mainly from Haverfordwest and occasionally from Pembroke or Neyland - show that, by the mid-eighteenth century, the situation had not altered to any great extent. By the early nineteenth century, however, larger ships were being built which were unable to reach Haverfordwest and Pembroke except at spring tides; silting of the channels was also becoming a problem. The newer towns, with greater depth of water available at their quays, began to take over more of the trade.

It was the larger vessels which traded further afield that were most affected by these changes. The smaller craft, carrying mainly coal and limestone, would have continued to ply their trade much as before. The fact that *Mary* had become a Pembroke Dock ship probably made little difference to her operations - in any case her days were numbered.

December was a time of the year when many of the coastal sloops had been laid up for the winter in one of the sheltered creeks of the Haven. But *Mary* was still at work. The westerly gale which sprang up on Sunday, 18th December, 1853, would have come as no surprise to her master John Percy, who dropped anchor in the lee of the cliffs to ride out the storm.

During the night the wind changed direction and began to blow a severe gale from the south-east. *Mary* was no longer protected from the fury of the storm; her anchor cables parted and she was driven out of the shelter of the Haven. Here *Mary* was at the mercy of wind and tide which bore her relentlessly towards Jack Sound and Skomer.

With its fierce currents and its submerged rocks, it is a treacherous place at the best of times. But, on this occasion. the ship had to contend with mountainous seas and a raging gale. And, perhaps mercifully, it was dark. To the terrified crew, the prospect of being dashed against the cliffs of Skomer or the mainland was perhaps even more frightening than the horrors of Jack Sound; in any case there was nothing they could do that would make any difference.

In the event it was in the heaving waters of Jack Sound that they found themselves. There was just a faint chance that the ship would be driven right through the sound. It was not to be. Suddenly she struck, and within minutes the sloop had been pounded to pieces. The crew must have thought their end had come. But the Fates relented on Captain Percy and his shipmates. *Mary* had not been cast up on the Black Stones or the Tusker - had she struck one of those wave-swept rocks there would have been no escape for those aboard the little ship.

Mary had, in fact, come ashore on Midland Island. Battered and bruised, soaked to the skin, the crew managed to fight their way through the surf and scramble onto firm ground. There, cold and hungry, they huddled together for warmth. And there, on the Tuesday morning, when the gale had subsided, they were found and rescued by the crew of a boat which had set out from nearby Marloes.

III; The Great Gale

The morning of Tuesday, 25th October, 1859, dawned fine and clear at Broad Haven. On the beach a grounded sloop was being loaded with culm. It was late in the season for a ship to be using this exposed bay, but *True Bess* was a St. David's vessel, and the relatively secure harbour of Porthclais was only a few miles distant across St. Bride's Bay.

True Bess, a 20 ton sloop built at Aberaeron in 1846, was originally one of several small vessels owned by Samuel Williams, merchant, of Rock House, St. David's. A familiar sight around the bay, she had been used for carrying culm and limestone for her owner who was, among other things, a coal merchant and lime burner.

Much of the culm came from Nolton, and account books of the Folkeston Colliery record that *True Bess* came here often in the late 1840s under her master David Williams, and that her cargo capacity was 30 tons. Folkeston Colliery was one of the principal mines of the St. Bride's Bay Coalfield, which stretched from Newgale in the north, through Nolton and Broad Haven, to Little Haven.

All four beaches were used to export the culm, but Nolton was by far the most important. Only here had any attempt been made to build a quay, though it offered little protection from the westerly gale. At all these places the ships were beached at high tide, then loaded from carts when the water receded. The trade was seasonal, most of the exports to destinations in Cardiganshire and North Pembrokeshire taking place between May and September.

But *True Bess* was not solely engaged in the local culm and limestone trade. Samuel Williams was a corn and general merchant who had wider interests. *True Bess* also traded with Bristol; in February, 1850, she arrived there with a cargo of 1220 barrels of barley from Solva.

In 1856 Samuel Williams sold his shipping interests and moved to Cardiff, and later to Liverpool where he set up as a ship broker. *True Bess* was purchased by John Davies, farmer, of Rhosson, near St. David's, who became a lime burner at Porthclais. He appointed Thomas Williams as master of the sloop.

So it happened that, on the fateful day, *True Bess* was loading culm at Broad Haven. During the day the weather began to deteriorate rapidly, and it became obvious that a severe storm was imminent. To remain where he was would be to court disaster, but the master had to wait for the incoming tide to float the ship off the beach.

By the time he was able to weigh anchor, the north-easterly gale had become too strong for him to attempt to reach Porthclais or Solva. Captain Williams realised that his only chance of saving the ship was to make for Milford, even though that meant passing through the dreaded Jack Sound.

Long before *True Bess* had reached the sound, the wind had backed north-west and increased still further, trapping the sloop within the bay. The ship was driven ever closer to the cliffs; there was no way of saving her. The crew, in a last desperate attempt to save themselves, took up their survival positions, hoping to cling to floating wreckage when the ship went ashore.

Soon, drifting helplessly, the little ship struck the rocks between Little Haven and nearby Musselwick. Within minutes she was "literally smashed to atoms" in the surf. By morning nothing remained but driftwood. The master had lashed himself to the mast, and his badly mutilated body, with the skull stove in, was picked up during the day. Of the mate and the boy who formed the remainder of the crew there was no trace.

A tragic story, but by no means unusual. Only the date is significant, for this was the storm which sank the *Royal Charter* off the coast of Anglesey. Described in the *Liverpool Telegraph* as ".... perhaps the greatest storm of the century ...." it led to the loss of over a hundred vessels around the coast.

According to the *Haverfordwest and Milford Haven Telegraph* of 2nd November, over a dozen vessels had been wrecked around Pembrokeshire, with considerable loss of life; many others had been damaged. They included (it was reported) three Aberystwyth ships; *Morning Star* on Cardigan Bar, *Bristol Trader* at Ceibwr and *Wave* on Linney Sands. Lost at Cwmyreglwys (where the church was destroyed by the waves) was *Mathildis* of New Quay, and near Fishguard the *Adeona* of Cardigan. At Newport the local smack *Friends* was torn from her moorings and wrecked, while at sea the Milford smack *Mary* was believed lost with all hands. And, although this was the most severe of all nineteenth century storms, it was but one of many.

The final cost of the storm, as far as local ships and seamen were concerned, proved to be even greater than at first feared. *Abeona*, wrecked near the Cow and Calf rocks in Fishguard Bay, was a 30 ton smack from Cardigan. Built at St. Dogmael's in 1852, she was wholly owned by William Stephens, slate merchant, of Llechryd. In view of the tragic events that occurred elsewhere on the North Pembrokeshire coast, her crew had a remarkable escape.

The Shipping Registers reveal that at least four other Cardiganshire ships had been lost, together with all members of their crews, along the lonely and perilous coast between Fishguard and Cardigan. Dashed to pieces against the rocks, their wreckage, and the bodies of their crews, were strewn for miles along the shoreline. However, the elderly Aberystwyth sloop *Bristol Trader* was not among the victims; she was to survive for five more years before being wrecked near Fishguard, where her Aberystwyth-born master and owner Richard Thomas had by then settled.

Bristol Trader had been confused with *Swansea Trader* of Borth, a 35 ton smack, built at Bideford in 1828; the register records the latter as having been lost off Dinas Head.

Two Aberystwyth-owned vessels were lost near Cardigan; the dandy *Margaret Lloyd* and the smack *Morning Star*. Two masts seen protruding above the waves near the river mouth belonged to the former; a dandy, like

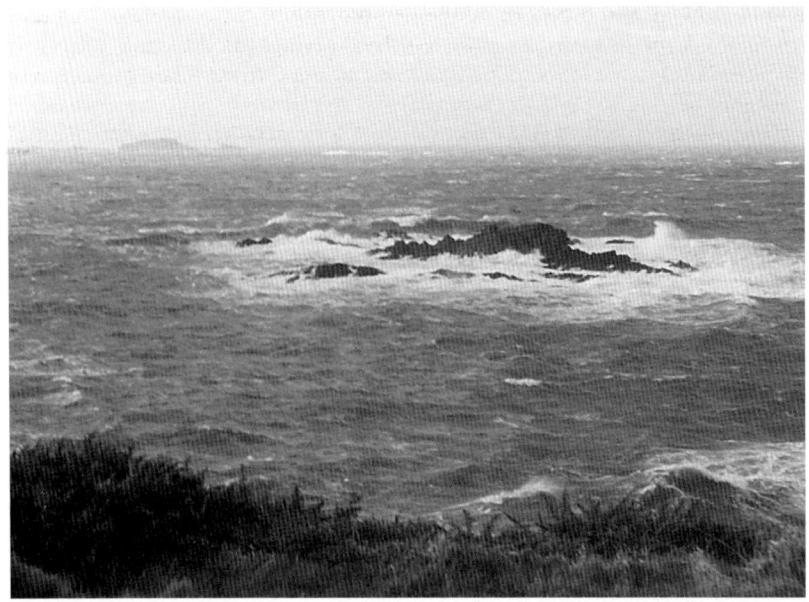

6. Carreg Gafeiliog, north of Ramsey Sound, during a winter gale, with North Bishop on horizon.

a ketch, has a short mizzen mast aft of the mainmast. *Margaret Lloyd*, a vessel of 53 tons and only five years old, had been lost together with all four members of her crew.

Cardigan Bar was given on the register as the site of the loss of the 47 ton Aberystwyth built *Morning Star*. At the time of her registration, ownership had been shared among nine persons, seven of whom came from Aberystwyth. Isaac Thomas (12 shares), John Thomas (10) and David Thomas (4) were all master mariners. Thomas Griffiths (14) was a maltster and Thomas Jones (4) a victualler; the representatives of Thomas Owen and Elizabeth Jones owned 10 and 4 shares respectively. Jane Thompson (2), widow, of Ludlow and Stephen Perkins (4) of Newport (Gwent) were the other owners.

Mathildis, wrecked near Cwmyreglwys with the loss of her crew of six was a 97 ton schooner belonging to New Quay. Lulled into setting sail by the previously calm weather she, like the others, had been trapped on a lee shore by the sudden northerly gale.

Further south on Linney Sands, near the mouth of the Haven, lay the remains of the 60 ton, three years old, Canadian built schooner *Wave* of Aberystwyth, laden with iron ore. Her crew also had perished, among them her owner and master John Hughes and his young son.

On one night five ships and over two dozen men from Aberystwyth, Borth and New Quay had been lost on the Pembrokeshire coast. It was a financial disaster for those who had invested their savings in the ships and their cargoes. But for the widows and children of the drowned sailors the future was grim indeed.

Few of the old time sailors have left first-hand accounts of experiences of storms such as that of 25th October, 1859. For the most part they were men of little formal education, but there was one, almost a century earlier, whose log survived; that man was Abel Hicks of Tremaenhir, near Solva.

During the 1760s Captain Hicks, according to Francis Green, was master, and probably part owner, of the 40 ton sloop *Industrious Bee*, whose chief owner was Richard Summers of Haverfordwest. In this small craft or in *Priscilla*, with a two-man crew, he traded regularly with Bristol. He also sailed to Liverpool, Belfast and Dublin, even to London, carrying culm from Little Milford, and corn and butter, mostly from Haverfordwest; returning with cargoes such as salt and tar and general merchandise.

On 6th February, 1761, Captain Hicks loaded a cargo of wheat, barley and oats at Haverfordwest. He made his way by stages down river to Angle, but bad weather delayed his departure. Almost a fortnight was to elapse before he was able to set sail from the Haven, on what was to prove a particularly hazardous voyage to Liverpool.

> "Wednesday the 18th. At 5 a clock in the morning unmored; no wind. Got under sail at 6 with lidle brees at W.S.W. At 9 got the harbour mouth with a Scotchman in company. At 12 the length of Scome. At 3 in the afternoon the length of the Bishops with fine brees at W.S.W.. At 6 Dinas Head bore E by S from us, 7 leags distand, wind at S.W., stout gale. At 12 at nite the Barges S.E. from us, 2 leags distand with a hard gale at S.W.. At 2 in the morning lowred down our main sail; at 3 took down our crogick went under bare powls for 3 houers blowing a great storm, the sea runing mountains heigh; shiped many turbulent seas; everything swiming on deck, raining and thick weather; could see no land; brote her head up under riff mainsail to lie to till would clear up; as she brote up shiped a terible sea over & over.
> At 7 a clock morninge Cleared up; we had Holyhead close on boord of us. At 8 the wind came to N.W.. Bore down to Dylas Bay. Came to at 12. Laid there 5 owars under a hard gale nite coming on, blowing like weather; got under sail and made for Blwmoris; got the river at 7 a clock at nite. Blowing like guns & snowing; could see nothing; got up to at 8. Laid there 2 days under blussterous weather. Sunday ye 22nd. Went under sail at 3 a clock in the morning, wind at S.W.. At 6 got the length of Worm's Head durty like weather. At 8 wind came to west, blowing hard; got over Chester Barr by 10; got Highlake at 11; got Liverpool at 2 in the afternoon. Blowing a perfect storm. Blessed be God that we are hear safe."

Captain Hicks had reason to give thanks for his safe arrival, as he did on many other occasions when he encountered gales on his voyages. Unlike many of his fellow captains he survived his career at sea, and eventually became a Commissioner for Land Tax and also part owner of Folkeston Colliery.

His survival owed much to his seamanship and to his profound knowledge of the seas he sailed; and no doubt to good fortune. Storms could spring up with little warning, and then all depended on a ship being able to reach a safe anchorage in time. Ability to foretell the weather was essential to the mariner, and this knowledge was handed down through the generations.

Fishguard Bay and Caldey Roads, near Tenby, were often used as shelter, but they were far from secure when the wind blew from the wrong quarter. There was talk, around 1800, of building a pier to enclose part of the bay to provide a harbour of refuge at Fishguard. It only came into being a century later with the construction of the breakwater by the Great Western Railway - long after the day of the coastal sailing ships.

Ships which could not reach port had to cope as best they could by seeking whatever shelter was available. One safe anchorage was in the lee of Ramsey Island, but it was a bold man who dared to enter the sound in a storm. Another refuge was Goultrop Roads in the south-eastern corner of St. Bride's Bay; but a change of wind brought oblivion to many a vessel sheltering there. It was at Goultrop that *True Bess* and her crew perished.

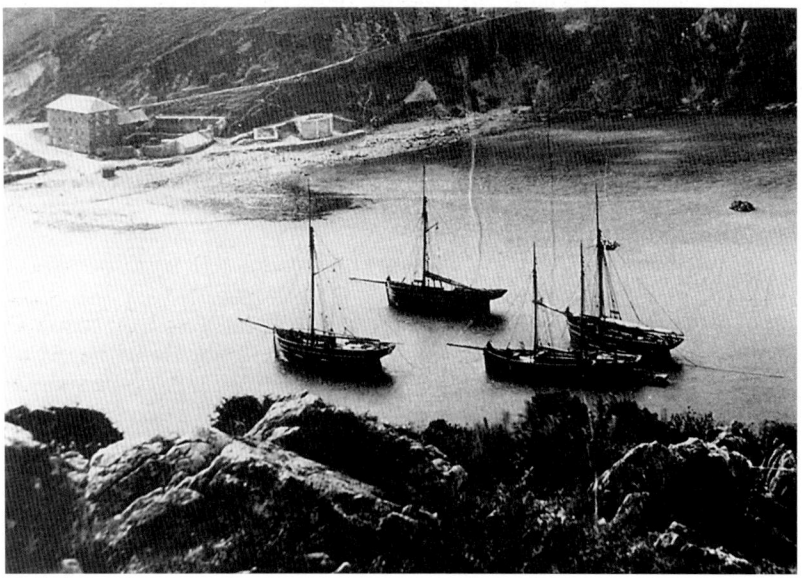

7. Three sloops and a small, two-masted schooner in the harbour of Lower Town, Fishguard; even here vessels were not secure during the worst storms.

IV; Collision Course

On the afternoon of 5th April, 1859, the smack *Mary* of St. Dogmael's was making her leisurely way down the winding estuary of the River Teifi. She was bound for Swansea with a cargo of flagstones. It was a voyage she was destined never to complete.

Mary had been built in 1842 at Glasson Dock, on the southern shore of the estuary of the River Lune in Lancashire; she had been registered at Lancaster on 1st November of that year. A 27 ton smack, 43 feet in length, she had operated from there for several years.

In 1850 she had been transferred to Cardigan and re-registered by her new owners, who all lived in St. Dogmael's. The largest holding was that of Thomas Davies, grocer, who owned 32 shares. The remaining 32 shares were held equally by two master mariners; David Davies and John Davies; the former became master of the vessel.

St. Dogmael's, northernmost of Pembrokeshire villages, stands on the left bank of the widening estuary of the Teifi a mile below Cardigan Bridge, the lowest crossing of the river. Cardigan itself was the port of register for the coast between Aberaeron and St. David's Head; in the nineteenth century the town was among the most important ports in Wales. Nearby St. Dogmael's shared in its prosperity.

As with other ports along Cardigan Bay, the bulk of the coastal trade involved the importation of culm and limestone, largely from Milford. The fertile Teifi valley produced considerable quantities of agricultural products, such as corn and butter, but, in common with most other ports along the coast, imports greatly exceeded exports.

There was, however, at least one other significant export. A few miles upstream, along the gorge at Cilgerran, were extensive slate quarries. The slates were loaded aboard barges, which carried them down river to Cardigan. Here they were transhipped to coastal sailing vessels such as *Mary* for distribution around the coast.

One of the vessels engaged in the slate trade was the 22 ton sloop *Ruby* of Cardigan which had been built there in 1839. Her owners were James and William Stephens, slate merchants of Llechryd, some four miles up the river from Cardigan. *Ruby* was one of the few local coasters to come to grief on the Bishops and Clerks. On 9th June, 1851, she was lost with all hands after being wrecked near the South Bishop.

The voyage from Cardigan to Swansea involved a long haul around the entire coast of Pembrokeshire with its many dangers. The first hazard, even before *Mary* had cleared harbour, would be the much-feared Cardigan Bar; a sandbank that lay across the mouth of the river. With the weather fair it should prove no obstacle to the experienced local mariner, but in adverse conditions it could be lethal. So it had proved on 30th September, 1841, to the sloop *Peggy* - whose owner and master was Thomas Davies of St.

Dogmael's - one of several ships from Cardigan and St. Dogmael's lost on the bar.

Once clear of the estuary, *Mary* would have set a course roughly west-south-west along the coast to St. David's Head. A hard and often barren shore; Cemaes Head, Dinas Head and Strumble Head; each posed its threat to the coastal sailor. *Union* of Cardigan had been lost near Cemaes Head on 10th November, 1866. But the bays could also prove dangerous; the 24 ton sloop *Providence* of Cardigan had been wrecked at Goodwick on 7th September, 1838, while the 23 ton *Jenny* of St. Dogmael's had been lost on 22nd October, 1840, at Newport.

After passing St. David's Head, the master would have altered course to take the *Mary* south on what was the most difficult and dangerous leg of the voyage. He would have had to navigate down Ramsey Sound with its numerous currents and counter-currents, then across St. Bride's Bay and finally through Jack Sound with its treacherous underwater rocks. Among the craft lost in this area were the St. Dogmael's sloops *Molly Lloyd*, wrecked on Ramsey Island on 15th September, 1842, and *Ann*, which was wrecked on 17th July, 1849, near Jack Sound.

The lighthouse on St. Ann's Head would have served as marker for those ships bound for Milford to alter course to enter the Haven. Some failed to make the entrance as did the 16 ton St. Dogmael's sloop *Morning Star*, which in May 1837 was: "lost at Blackpool near Milford Harbour."

When bound for Saundersfoot to load coal, or, as on her present voyage to Swansea, *Mary* would not change course to the east until she was clear of Linney Head. She would then have sailed along the isolated south coast, with its vertical limestone cliffs, as far as Caldey, before striking out across Carmarthen Bay for the south coast of Gower and, eventually, Swansea. There were fewer losses along this coast, but they included the St. Dogmael's sloop *Retriever*, wrecked on 15th October, 1869, at Old Castle Head, near Tenby, after striking rocks on St. Margaret's Island. Her master James Owen and crew landed by ship's boat at Lydstep.

It was none of these natural hazards that caused the loss of the *Mary*. Sailing along the north coast of Pembrokeshire, she was heading into the wind, so that *Mary* was obliged to tack alternately to port and starboard to progress along the coast.

About 10 p.m. she was on the port tack off Strumble Head. Suddenly, out of the darkness, another ship loomed. There was no time to take evasive action, in any case the broad-beamed sloops were slow to respond to the helm, and the other vessel struck *Mary* broadside on, tearing a deep gash in her side.

It was obvious that *Mary* had been badly damaged and was taking in water rapidly. The other vessel, the Cardigan sloop *Tivy*, was not seriously damaged by the collision. Fortunately *Mary* remained afloat long enough for her crew to scramble aboard the other sloop before their own sank. The survivors were then taken back to Cardigan aboard the *Tivy*.

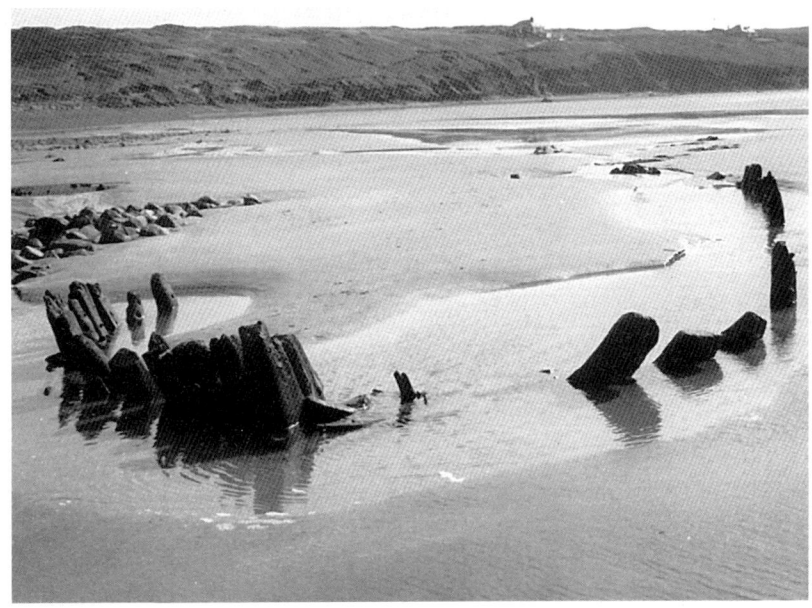

8. Wreck of small coastal trader exposed by winter storm at Whitesands, possibly *Bolina* of Bideford.

Some fifteen years later another Cardigan-registered *Mary* was the victim of a collision; this time with fatal consequences. A 23 ton sloop, built at Cardigan in 1837, her ownership was shared among eleven persons from Cardigan and the surrounding area; at the time of her loss, the managing owner was Mary Owen of the White Lion, Aberporth. During the early part of 1874 she had made a total of eight voyages bringing coal or culm from Hook, Pembrey and Llanelli, and limestone from Pembroke, Lydstep and Croft to Aberporth, Tresaith and Llangrannog, as well as to Cardigan itself.

The Dewsland and Kemes Guardian of 25th July, 1874, carried a report that the Great Western Railway steamer *Milford*, on passage from Waterford, had run down an unknown sloop at 1 a.m. the previous Thursday near St. Ann's Head. The report continued:

> "It was dark and cloudy at the time and nothing was seen of the vessel until the crash was heard. A boat was lowered but not a vestige of the vessel or its hapless crew could be seen, therefore the name of the vessel is at present unknown."

Some days later, the body of the master, David James, was recovered near the entrance to the Haven, and the identity of the sloop was established. Both master and mate, Morgan Jones, came from Cardigan; the body of the latter was not recovered.

Shortly before 4 a.m. on 30th September, 1873, another Aberporth owned vessel was run down off St. Ann's Head by the railway steamer *Great Western*. She was the 44 ton smack *Penrhyn Castle* which was apparently showing no lights. A boat lowered by the steamer succeeded in picking up two of the crew, though one later died. The survivor was the master John James; the boy Griffith Griffiths was drowned, while the mate Thomas James died of exhaustion.

The *Pembrokeshire Herald* of 6th February, 1856, describes how the *Perseverance* of Milford had run down a smack (named as the *Ann* of Cardigan) about 4 a.m. on a dark and stormy night during the previous week. The collision had taken place 4 miles off the South Bishop; two of the crew of the smack escaping by jumping aboard the larger vessel; the third Evan Rees was drowned. Newspaper reports, though descriptive, often contain errors concerning ships; in this case it is the name which is incorrect, the victim being the *Ann Jones* of St. Dogmael's. The entry in the register merely states 'run down off Milford.'

The advent of steamships brought a greatly increased danger of collision, particularly at night or in fog which sometimes blanketed the coast. The sloops really belonged to another age, when most of the traffic consisted of cumbersome, slow-moving craft like themselves. At night, their lights would have been provided by, at best, oil lamps, which could be seen far enough away for avoiding action to be taken.

The steamships were much larger, generally built of iron, and travelled at high speeds even in poor visibility. The sloops would have had little time to take action to avoid the swiftly moving steamers. To save time and fuel, the steamers were apt to take short cuts through the sounds, waters normally avoided by the large sailing ships, bringing them into the channels used by the coastal traders. Speed was essential to the steamships; the number which ran headlong into cliffs such as Linney Head suggests that they did not themselves always keep an adequate lookout.

The crew of a sloop which was run down by a steamer would have a poor chance of survival. There would be little time for them to escape from the sinking ship, and, even if the steamer did stop and make a search, it was unlikely that the survivors could be found in time. The crew of the *Mary* of St. Dogmael's were indeed fortunate that the vessel which came out of the night was only another sloop.

V; The Final Straw

The bows of the little smack alternately rose and dipped as she butted her way northwards through Ramsey Sound on Wednesday, 4th September, 1861. To observers on the shore she seemed to be riding low in the water; the smack was obviously heavily laden. Again her bows dipped, but this time they did not rise, and, in view of the horrified watchers, she vanished beneath the waves, carrying her crew with her.

Although the unfortunate vessel could not be immediately identified, her description fitted that of the 19 ton smack *Rechabite* of Fishguard, which failed to arrive as expected at her home port. A report, dated 20th September, in the *Pembrokeshire Herald* confirmed that the casualty was indeed the *Rechabite*, which had been bound for Fishguard with a cargo of culm from the south of the county.

The report stated that there had been two men on board the missing vessel; Levi Davies, the master, who also owned the smack, and John Llywellyn, the mate. The latter left a widow with several small children to bring up; an ordeal faced by many wives and families of the old time sailors, in days when state aid was unknown.

In Fishguard there was much talk about the reasons for the loss of the vessel, and the finger was pointed at her owner. Levi Davies was accused of overloading the ship; the feelings in the locality were reported in the *Pembrokeshire Herald:*

> "The untimely fate of these men should serve as a warning to masters of coastal vessels, against taking in too large a cargo. An opinion is very general in this neighbourhood that the little vessel was overloaded at the time she disappeared beneath the water."

The local seafarers would have known their facts. They would have been aware of the cargo which each of the local vessels could safely carry, and they could have identified those masters who exceeded that limit. Very likely the disaster had been predicted.

If those who saw the disaster take place thought the smack looked familiar, it would hardly have been surprising. *Rechabite*, built at Lawrenny in 1840, had originally been a St. David's vessel. Her principal owners had been Ebenezer Williams, draper, and his brother Samuel, merchant, each of whom held sixteen shares. William Richards, master mariner (who later sold his shares to the brothers) and Ebenezer Rees of Croeswdig, farmer, both owned eight shares, while the remaining owners; John Mortimer of Treginnis, farmer, Thomas Lewis of Dyffryn, farmer, Blanch Maria Davies of Carnachenwen, widow, and John Howells of Solva, innkeeper, held four shares apiece. All, apart from the last three, came from St. David's town or parish.

Multiple ownership of even small vessels, with the shares held by eight or more persons, was common in Cardiganshire and North Pembrokeshire during the first half of the nineteenth century. The 35 ton smack *Mary Jane* of New Quay (lost off the Isle of Man in 1863) had no fewer than thirty joint owners. Farmers and merchants or shopkeepers were the most important owners, together with mariners (especially the master) and sometimes the shipbuilder. And there were many others; carpenters, coopers and maltsters, widows and spinsters, as well as the gentry, who owned shares in one or more ships.

During the 1840s, *Rechabite* spent most of her time carrying culm and limestone to Porthclais for Samuel Williams. The records of Folkeston Colliery show that the vessel made a number of voyages from Nolton to St. David's carrying a maximum of 30 tons of culm. There were a few voyages to Goodwick with culm for Thomas Lewis, who was one of the local lime burners. For these the load was only 28 tons, perhaps in recognition of the much more hazardous nature of the longer voyage through Ramsey Sound and along the north coast past Strumble Head to Goodwick.

According to *Slater's Directory*, in 1850 *Rechabite* was one of three ships which operated as Bristol Traders from Solva and St. David's on a monthly basis. Particularly during the winter months they carried corn, and during February 1850, *Rechabite* was one of no fewer than six ships which sailed to Bristol with cargoes of wheat, barley and oats; in her case the cargo was 1,240 bushels of barley. No doubt, the higher prices which could be obtained during winter months made these stormy passages worth the risks involved.

On 22nd December, 1854, Samuel Williams mortgaged his 20 shares in *Rechabite* to William Walters, banker, of Haverfordwest; this was later discharged. Ebenezer Williams died in 1856, but the only further entry in the register notes the loss of the vessel. Samuel Williams, in his list of shipwrecks, confirms that *Rechabite* then belonged to Fishguard. However, there is no record of when Levi Davies purchased his shares, or of how many he owned.

On 8th October, 1864, a sloop called *Little Neptune* of Aberporth suffered a similar fate. Too heavily laden (it was reported) for the sea conditions at the time, she foundered in Broad Sound - between Skomer and Skokholm - with the loss of all three crew members.

The first half of the nineteenth century was a period of relative prosperity for agriculture in West Wales. Its success depended upon the availability of lime to neutralize the acid soils of the area. Many small sloops were built to carry the culm and limestone required to produce the lime. The limekilns where the process was carried out are still to be seen at virtually every creek and beach where the sloops could be run ashore to discharge their cargoes.

After 1850 there was a decline in agriculture. In addition, more effective fertilizers were becoming available. Fewer ships were needed to transport the culm and limestone. Ships were lost, others lay rotting on mud banks. Those that survived had to work even harder to make a profit in an ever increasing recession. Times were hard and economies had to be made.

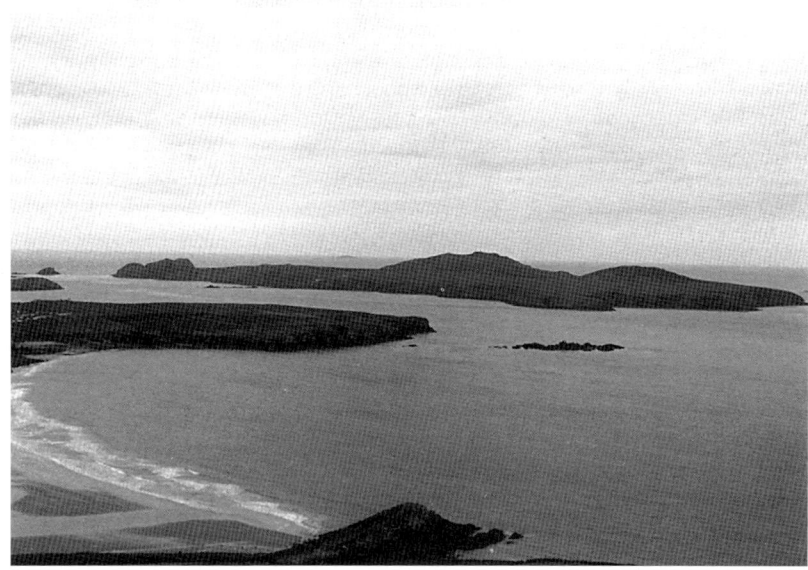

9. Ramsey Island, with Ramsey Sound and the Bitches, viewed from the slopes of Carnllidi; Grassholm on horizon to left of higher hill.

The owners of the Milford cutter *Antelope* decided to convert her for oyster fishing. On 25th November, 1875, she was engaged in this pursuit in St. Bride's Bay when she sprang a leak and foundered at Goultrop Roads. Her hull was not seriously damaged and she was later, after several attempts, raised with the help of two large smacks. However she does not seem to have been put back into service.

One way to economise was to reduce manpower. Traditionally the crew of a coastal smack had been "two men and a boy"; the latter could be as young as eleven years of age. With the experience he gained he later became the mate and - if he survived - eventually the master. But by the second half of the century, the crew was normally just master and mate or even master and boy.

There was one man who went even further. He was W. P. Ormond of Old Bridge, Haverfordwest (coal, corn and flour merchant) the owner of the small smack *Alice*. Her master, and at times sole member of the crew was George Brace.

On the morning of Monday, 20th September, 1880, *Alice*, with a cargo of limestone, was beating down the Haven against a stiff breeze and strong tide. About eleven o'clock, when opposite Pembroke Gut, she suddenly vanished leaving a cask and other floating wreckage to mark the spot where she had sunk; but of the one man aboard there was no trace. The suddenness of the sinking was attributed to the nature of the cargo; but the fact that there was no mate to help in handling the sails must have been significant. A fortnight later, a body, fully clothed "with the exception of the hat", was washed ashore near Angle. It was believed to be that of the missing master.

The *Lady of the Lake* of Milford, carrying limestone from Lydstep to Tenby, also had only one man aboard when she foundered near Bear Cave on 11th May, 1870; the solitary seaman escaped in the ship's boat. Probably too small to be registered, *Lady of the Lake* was the third vessel employed by the contractors at St. Catherine's Fort to be lost within a period of less than two years.

Some owners attempted to increase their profits by taking on extra cargo. In early Victorian times there were no regulations concerning the loading of ships, and many put to sea in a grossly overloaded condition. It was not until 1876 that the Merchant Shipping Act, promoted by Samuel Plimsoll, came into effect and put an end to this practice.

In any case the typical broad-beamed sloop had little enough freeboard (often one foot or less) even when loaded normally. On 1st September, 1843, in poor visibility, the Bristol paddle-steamer *Queen* ran onto rocks off Skokholm Island and began to sink. Fortunately, becalmed nearby was the sloop *Hope* of Abercastle laden with limestone. The survivors were transferred to the sloop but, before they could be taken on board, the master, David Jenkins, was forced to jettison much of the cargo, otherwise the *Hope* herself would have been in danger of sinking.

It was providential that the sloop was in the vicinity, or there would have been many more casualties than the one fatality. Even aboard the *Hope* the survivors were not entirely safe as she drifted with the currents; only many hours later, when the fog had lifted, did David Jenkins dare make for harbour at Milford.

Levi Davies, as owner and master of the *Rechabite* needed to make a profit. To this end he employed only one other man as crew, and for the shorter voyages the two could probably have coped satisfactorily. But he also saw the advantage of carrying as much cargo as he possibly could; and that was to prove his undoing.

Ramsey Sound often looks placid enough, but the currents which sweep through it are lethal. The immediate cause of the sinking of *Rechabite* is unknown, but it was undoubtedly those last few cartloads of culm that killed Levi Davies and the mate.

VI; Crossing the Bar

Among the ships included on the Cardigan register in the mid-nineteenth century was the sloop *Taff of Twenty Two*. Her curious name probably arose from the fact that she was built in Cardiff in 1822, and it served to distinguish her from other ships named after that river.

Her early years were presumably spent working out of Cardiff, but on 21st August, 1827, she was registered anew at Cardigan. The principal shareholder was her master, William Rees of Dinas. who owned thirty six shares; the remainder were held by another mariner and a widow from Dinas, a sailmaker and a ropemaker from Fishguard, and a lock-keeper from Cardiff who had probably been one of the original owners.

On 17th February, 1835, William Rees was replaced as master by George Williams, also of Dinas. On 28th February, the former disposed of all but eight of his shares in the sloop to four other persons. On the same date, two of the other previous owners sold their shares to a farmer and a shopkeeper.

Later there were other minor changes in ownership. Then on 15th March, 1845, *Taff of Twenty Two* was re-registered at Cardigan. Five of the owners were mariners; George Williams, her master, held eight shares, as did William Rees, the former master; David Rees, Thomas Llewellyn of Penrhiw and David Evans of Cwmbach each held four shares. All five were from the parish of Dinas. There were two widows; Margaret Griffiths of Trewrach and Anne Williams of Dinas, owners of four and eight shares respectively; and a farmer, George Davies of Tyllwyd, who owned four shares. Two men from Fishguard; William Williams, ropemaker and Thomas Francis, shipwright, held eight shares apiece. Finally John Morgan 'locker' of Cardiff retained the remaining four shares.

Though much smaller than either Fishguard or Newport and with no proper harbour, Dinas was equally involved in maritime affairs. The multiple ownership of *Taff of Twenty Two* is typical, with owners coming from the seafaring, shipbuilding and farming communities. In the larger towns merchants and shopkeepers were important, but in the case of *Taff of Twenty Two* they had only one representative - James Harries, shopkeeper, of Bwlchyrhos, Dinas, who between 1835 and 1840 held four shares.

Taff of Twenty Two presumably spent much of her time carrying culm and limestone to North Pembrokeshire. But, in all probability, her main base was Fishguard. According to the *Carmarthen Journal*, on 10th June, 1839, two Fishguard sloops, *Taff* and *Hazard*, collided during a thunderstorm; the former towed the more seriously damaged *Hazard* to safety at Hubberston. On 25th March, 1850, the Bristol Trade Presentments record the arrival from Fishguard of the *Taff*, master G. Williams, with 29 sacks and 200 quarters of oats. Altogether during the year a total of eleven cargoes carried in six different ships arrived from Fishguard; with one exception they included corn, almost exclusively oats.

In October 1851 her travels took *Taff of Twenty Two* to Cardigan. To reach the quay, ships had to thread their way upstream along the winding channel between the shifting sandbanks. Most notorious of these was the Cardigan Bar which lay across the mouth of the river. It is a hazardous spot, particularly when the incoming tide meets the river in spate, turning the estuary into a seething mass of foam. Under such conditions, the slightest error in judgement can be disastrous. Her master made such an error and *Taff of Twenty Two* struck the sandbank where she was pounded to pieces in the surf.

It was above all the bar which restricted the growth of Cardigan as a port, and many vessels were wrecked there. A sandbank across the mouth of the River Nevern hindered the development of Newport - its victims included the Cardigan-registered sloop *Royal Oak*, wrecked on the beach during May 1865. The harbour at Lower Town, Fishguard, had no such restrictions and became the chief harbour of North Pembrokeshire.

The problem at Solva was different. Here the main approach to the harbour lay between two jagged reefs - Black Rock to the west and St. Elvis Rock to the east. In rough weather it is an awesome sight, with the boiling surf surging through the narrow gap, a terrifying prospect for the homecoming mariner. In order to make it more visible at night, the Black Rock was, on 3rd July, 1882, painted white with lime - an event recorded in the *Haverfordwest and Milford Haven Telegraph*. Surprisingly, apart from an unnamed vessel loaded with slate listed by Samuel Williams as being wrecked on Black Rock, there seem to be no recorded instances of shipwrecks at the entrance to Solva Harbour.

The Solva smack *Water Lily* had an extremely lucky escape in May 1900 after running aground on the Black Rock. Attempts by her master and owner Henry John to refloat her using a kedge failed and it was feared she would capsize when the tide receded. However by good fortune the smack had grounded on a flat surface; she was refloated on the next tide after part of her cargo had been jettisoned.

The narrow harbour entrance at Porthclais, some four miles to the west, claimed the 21 ton smack *Courier* (or *Le Courier*) in 1879. Built at Hakin in 1859, she was first registered in the name of John Thomas of Hakin. He shortly afterwards mortgaged the ship to William Walters of Haverfordwest. Walters. who had premises in High Street, was one of the leading bankers in the area, and frequently lent money using ships as security. On 21st December, 1859, while the ship was at Milford, a fire broke out in the cabin, threatening to spread to the cargo of coal from Cardiff. Due to the quick reactions of the owner's workmen it was extinguished, though not before causing considerable damage to the decks and cabin.

During the following year, *Courier* was sold to Alexander McKay of Point Street, Hakin, who immediately raised a mortgage of £70, at interest of £5 per cent per annum on the ship. Some time later, the ship was sold to William Williams, merchant, of Grove Hotel, St. David's.

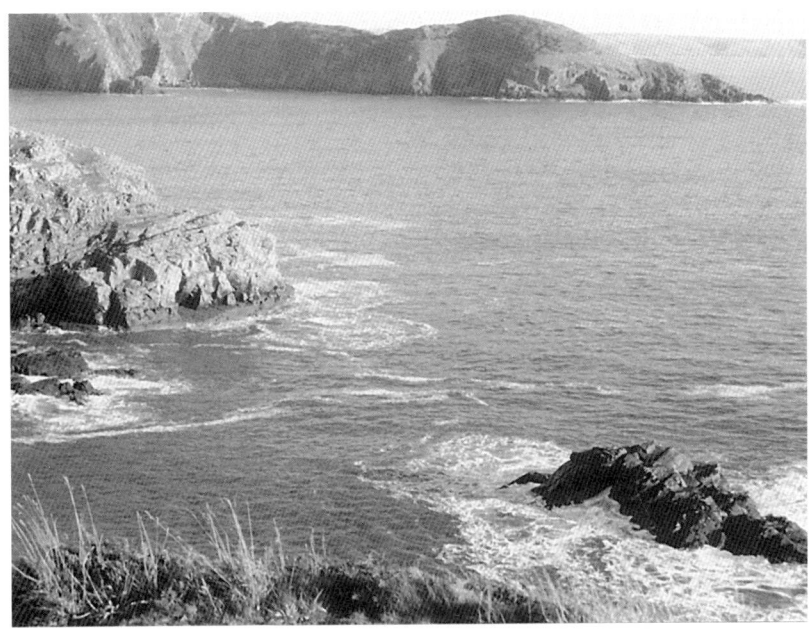

10. The narrow and hazardous entrance to Solva Harbour, with St. Elvis Rock on left and Black Rock (Carreg Ddu) on right.

During 1879, her final year, *Courier* had made nine voyages with limestone and six with culm from Milford to St. David's, as well as two with culm from Little Haven and one with coal from Porthcawl. She had also made two voyages to Swansea carrying barley, returning with coal.

On 18th October, George Lile, her master, was attempting to take *Courier*, carrying culm from Little Haven, through the narrow channel past the breakwater at Porthclais. While making her approach she "missed her stays", failing to alter course and running onto the rocks, where she became a total loss. The master and mate - William Mortimer - contrived, with difficulty, to escape in the small boat. George Lile lived at Penporthclais, which overlooked the harbour entrance, and undoubtedly his waiting family provided an audience for his misfortune.

On 3rd August, 1868, the smack *Pearl* - owned by George Thomas of Pembroke, Government contractor for St. Catherine's Fort at Tenby - was discharging a cargo of limestone at the island quay. During the evening a north-easterly gale sprang up, putting the vessel in some danger. About 9 p.m., as the crew was attempting to haul the craft off to come into the harbour, the rope parted and she was driven onto the rocks on the point; as she drifted her mast struck the suspension bridge to the island causing considerable damage to the structure. The crew fortunately escaped in the ship's boat, but *Pearl* became a total loss.

Pearl had run aground before, on 18th December, 1853, while sheltering from a gale near Saundersfoot. Her crew had taken refuge in the rigging, and had only been rescued by the bravery of Thomas Noot who had swum out from the shore with a rope. Brand new, *Pearl* had been worth the strenuous and lengthy effort required to refloat her.

In September 1869, *Morning Star*, owned by her elderly master Thomas James of Milford, was loading sand at Tenby South Beach in connection with the contract for the Fort. A change in wind direction drove her further up the beach where she was broken up by the gale which developed.

While attempting to enter Saundersfoot Harbour on 5th November, 1854, the sloop *Nautilus* of Laugharne ran aground. According to the *Haverfordwest and Milford Haven Telegraph* of 11th November she was expected to become a total wreck. However the *Pembrokeshire Herald*, published the previous day, announced she had been refloated with little damage. *Nautilus* continued to ply her trade for many more years until, in 1926, after nearly ninety years service, she was converted to river use only.

St. Ann's Head, guardian of the entrance to Milford Haven, is named after the medieval chapel dedicated to St. Ann which once stood on the point. It provided a marker for ships entering the Haven; it was later replaced by two lighthouses which were rebuilt about 1800. Even so the opening in the cliffs could be difficult to pick out, and losses continued to occur.

Probably the greatest disaster in the days of sail occurred on the night of Saturday, 10th September, 1866. Seven or eight large sailing ships, running before a gale in driving rain which limited visibility, attempted to enter the Haven. The leading vessel ran aground near St. Ann's. The remainder, following the leader, were all wrecked in what became known as the 'Mill Bay Disaster'. Loss of life was heavy, and matched only by the tragic sinking of two landing craft during the Second World War.

Wrecks involving the coastal sloops were much less spectacular and costly in terms of life. But, over the years, the approaches to the Haven claimed many victims among the local traders.

One of the vessels lost nearby was the Fishguard sloop *Fidelity*. Built in 1807, her last registry was at Cardigan on 9th January, 1826. Her owners at that time were: David Stephens, sailmaker (12 shares), William Hughes, currier (5), William Meyler, farmer (10), William Williams, ropemaker (10) and Mary Ann Lloyd, widow (13). All five lived in Fishguard. There were two owners from Llanychaer; John Lewis, farmer (10) and Elizabeth Lewis, spinster (1). The remaining 3 shares were listed as 'Fractions'.

On the night of 21st July, 1846, *Fidelity* was on passage to Milford. When nearing St. Ann's Head she failed to go about, and drifted ashore about a mile north of the lighthouse. The two men aboard escaped by clambering along the bowsprit to reach the rocks and then climbing the cliffs. They made their way to the lighthouse, where they were given food and shelter, before continuing their journey on foot to Milford. Within a few hours *Fidelity* became a total wreck.

The *Pembrokeshire Herald* of 27th November, 1863, reported the remarkable rescue of the crew of a smack which failed to make the entrance to Milford Haven in gale-force winds. The vessel was identified as *Eleanor Grace* of Llanelli - a 27 ton smack, built at Landshipping in 1834. She was strictly no longer a Llanelli ship, having been purchased by her master, Charles Hunt of Bridgwater. However, she continued to operate largely from Llanelli, and was on this occasion sailing to Pembroke Dock with a cargo of coal.

About 11 a.m. on Saturday 21st November, a Mr. Roach of Linney observed *Eleanor Grace* rounding Linney Head in a sinking condition. Realising she had no chance of making the Haven entrance, he sent a man on horseback the eight miles to Bosherston to summon the coastguards with their life-saving apparatus.

The stricken ship dropped anchor in the cove known as Bluckspool, but the seas swept away the small boat before it could be launched. Soon afterwards the smack sank and the crew of two men and a boy took to the rigging as she began to break up. There, drenched by the waves, they clung on desperately until about 3.45 p.m. when at last the coastguards arrived on the scene.

There was no time to be lost; the mortar was quickly set up, and a line fired towards the ship. The first shot fell short; the second reached its target, but the men failed to grasp the line. Coastguard E. Lewis, at great peril to himself, scrambled across the wave-swept rocks to shout instructions to the men. This done, with great difficulty he regained the shore. A third shot was fired. This was successful and the three were soon brought ashore before being taken to Linney for food and rest.

On 8th January, 1864, a somewhat different account, based on the report of PC Griffiths, appeared. According to this, it was he who had persuaded Mr Roach (who had considered it a pointless exercise) to send for the coastguards. Mr Roach had then gone off for his dinner, leaving the constable alone at the scene. Only when the coastguards arrived, had Mr Roach reappeared.

To the crew of *Eleanor Grace*, like those of *Fidelity*, *Taff* and *Courier*, it was a case of so near and yet so far. They were so nearly home; but the last mile could sometimes be the most dangerous of all. They were lucky and escaped with their lives. Many were less fortunate.

Doubly fortunate were Levi Harries and his crew. On 22nd August, 1868, the smack *Ellen Gwenllian*, owned by Robert Morgan, merchant, of Haverfordwest, but then trading from Fishguard, was lost near the entrance to Milford Haven. Levi Harries, Richard Thomas and Thomas Owen were all saved. Only weeks previously, on 21st July, the same three men had been rescued when the Fishguard smack *Curlew*, of which Levi Harries was managing owner, had foundered.

VII; No Hiding Place

The restless sea which sculpted the serrated Pembrokeshire coast gave it one priceless asset - its harbours. Long narrow inlets sheltered by hills, the drowned mouths of its rivers provide safe anchorage in all but the worst of weathers. Best by far is the magnificent expanse of Milford Haven, nearly twenty miles in length from St. Ann's Head to Haverfordwest, with many landlocked creeks and roadsteads where hundreds of ships could ride at anchor. But by its very size it could sometimes turn into a death trap should the wind change suddenly. So it proved on 1st February, 1876, to the smack *Ant*.

Of 27 tons register and 41 feet in length, *Ant* had been built in 1827 at Milford by William Roberts, one of a well known local family of shipbuilders. She was obviously built as a speculative venture; for some time no purchaser came forward, and William Roberts, whose place of residence was in Hakin, operated the craft himself.

The shipyard owned by the Roberts brothers was on the Milford shore of what was then the tidal Hubberston Pill, near the end of the present Victoria Bridge. During the early years of the nineteenth century they built a considerable number of vessels, mainly sloops, in many cases retaining shares in the vessel.

Though few details are known of her early career, *Ant* apparently traded with Ireland, as her original master, Henry Morgan, was replaced by John Morgan (a native of Solva) at Waterford on 8th October, 1830. Pigot in 1835 described *Ant* as a coastal trader and listed her among the vessels trading between Haverfordwest, Milford and Bristol.

By then William Roberts had succeeded in selling a half share in the smack, by Bill of Sale dated 3rd August, 1831. The purchaser was Joseph Tombs of Haverfordwest, who owned shares in a number of vessels. In the 1830 edition of the *Directory of South Wales* he is described as grocer of Quay Street. By the 1835 edition he had become tallow chandler, butter merchant and factor, as well as grocer; his premises were situated on both sides of Quay Street at its junction with High Street.

Tombs was a man of enterprise; it was he, together with Captain Thomas Richards of Haverfordwest and Thomas Corey, a Bristol merchant, who was responsible for purchasing the new 110 ton paddle-steamer *County of Pembroke*. In all some twenty six persons were involved, eighteen of whom were from Pembrokeshire, including thirteen from Haverfordwest; the remainder came from Bristol.

The vessel replaced the ill-fated paddle-steamer *Frolic*, which had established the Haverfordwest - Bristol route in 1830. *Frolic* had been wrecked on Nash Sands on 16th March, 1831; there were no survivors. Sadly, *County of Pembroke*, the only significant locally-owned paddle-steamer to operate the route, proved financially unsuccessful, and was sold to Bristol owners in 1833. However, the service continued under Bristol ownership for a number of years using a variety of ships.

In 1835 *County of Pembroke*, under her new owners, was again on the Bristol run. Steam had not yet killed off the sailing ships on the route; seven of these being described as 'Bristol Traders', although the steamers had creamed off the passenger traffic. The reign of the passenger steamers was short, being brought to an end by the coming of the railway in 1853, though they continued to carry cargo on the route for many years.

Although a few sailing vessels continued to ply fairly regularly between Haverfordwest and Bristol until the 1850s, they were a dying breed. Joseph Tombs must have realised this, and on 14th May, 1838, he disposed of his shares in *Ant* to Margaret Roberts, widow, administratrix of the late William Roberts. Mrs. Roberts, who then lived in Milford, became sole owner and continued to operate the smack for almost a decade.

In 1847 *Ant* was sold outside the Haven for the first time. Her new owners were John Williams, merchant, of Solva, and his master mariner namesake. The former was owner of some half dozen sloops, which were used largely in connection with the considerable lime burning business he carried out in Solva. Mr. Williams prospered greatly, and was responsible for building the imposing Tanyrallt in Lower Solva; he also constructed the impressive adjacent granary. For a quarter of a century he operated *Ant* profitably, employing her almost entirely in the culm and limestone trade.

By 1872 Benjamin Vaughan was master; the crew of three included his thirteen years old son and namesake. During the first half of the year, *Ant* made one voyage each from Saundersfoot and Nolton with culm and ten from Milford with culm and limestone; between July and December there were a further eleven voyages from Milford - all with limestone. But the writing was on the wall. Two years later *Ant*, which carried about 32 tons of cargo, was down to a total of thirteen voyages from Milford to Solva, though she still carried a crew of three.

On 21st December, 1874, *Ant* was sold to William Jenkins, shipwright, and John Thomas, shoemaker, both of St. Ishmael's. So *Ant* returned to the Haven which had been her birthplace and from which she had sailed for two decades. It was not to be a happy return. Barely a year later, on 1st February, 1876, a winter storm drove *Ant* ashore at Sandy Haven, the creek nearest to St. Ishmael's, with the result that she became a total loss.

Another vessel wrecked in Sandy Haven was the Aberystwyth-registered sloop *Betsey* which was lost on 5th May, 1829, in strange circumstances. Under her master John Morgan she had been carrying culm from Saundersfoot to Aberdyfi when she was in collision with the sloop *John* of Fishguard (master John Jones) some three miles off St. Ann's Head.

Fearing *Betsey* was about to sink, the crew took to their small boat and landed safely at Dale. The abandoned vessel however remained afloat and was carried by wind and tide into the Haven, eventually drifting ashore at Sandy Haven and being broken up by the gale which developed.

By no means all the accidents which took place in harbour could be attributed to nature; many were due to human error. One day in July 1862, the smack *Ann* of Cardigan was moored in Castle Pill, Milford Haven. As the tide receded she settled on her anchor which pierced her bottom, causing her to sink in shallow water.

Ann was refloated as were several other vessels which sank in the Haven, some of which had been written off. The smack *Britannia* of St. Dogmael's was (according to the Cardigan Register) "totally lost at Lawrenny Reach 29 Nov. 1862. This vessel was sold as a total wreck, and on restoration to seaworthiness registered anew." *Britannia*, then owned by Richard Evans of Borth and registered at Aberystwyth, had previously been stranded at Ceibwr during the great gale of October, 1859. Twice salvaged and repaired, her remarkable career ended in August, 1881, when, as the Milford registered *Britannia* of Dinas, she was lost off St. David's Head.

In the confined and congested waters of Milford Haven collisions were bound to happen. On 25th November, 1838, the large sloop *Industry* of Aberystwyth was "run foul of by another vessel" and sank at Musselwick near Dale Roads. The wreck was purchased by Captain John Morgans of St. David's and raised in the following June. Structural damage was less severe than was first thought and, after extensive repairs, *Industry* was re-registered at Milford.

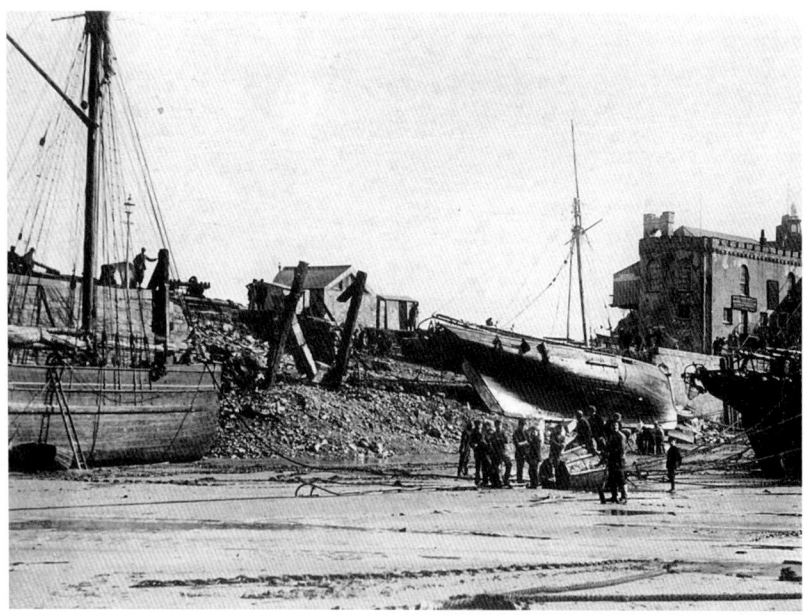

11. Aftermath of storm of 20th October, 1896, at Tenby Harbour, as a result of which the cutter *Wasp* became a total loss.

Greatly feared by the sailor was fire. On 4th January, 1876, the Aberystwyth-registered, though by then locally-owned, smack *Catherine* caught fire at Porthclais and became a total loss. Some months later her master, Samuel Prosser, was awarded compensation of £2.15.0 by the grandly named 'Shipwrecked Fishermen and Mariners Royal Benevolent Fund' for the loss of his clothing. Luckily, the blaze happened in harbour and not at sea where the crew would have been in mortal danger.

Another victim of fire was the smack *Wave Queen* (master Fred Vittle of the Royal George, Pembroke) owned by Ann Vittle of Robert Street, Milford. Up to 30th May, when she was burnt out, she had spent most of 1893 trading within Milford Haven. Her crew also escaped with their lives.

Nevertheless, even in harbour the greatest danger was the sea itself. During the Great Gale of 25th October, 1859, two sloops - *Lilly* and *Jane* - broke adrift in Fishguard Harbour and were driven against the ramshackle old bridge over the Gwaun, causing its partial collapse. On that occasion Solva escaped the worst, but a week later, with the wind in the opposite direction, many ships sheltering there were battered by a second severe storm.

On the latter occasion the smack *Eagle*, with a cargo of culm from Swansea for Aberaeron, had taken shelter in the Haven. She parted her cables and was carried against Milford Pier where she was scuttled to avoid further damage. A second smack the *Eliza* of Haverfordwest, in ballast for Porthcawl, also broke adrift and was driven against the partly submerged *Eagle*. Both smacks were reported to be total losses and the pier was badly damaged; neither vessel was insured.

One of the most destructive storms inside Milford Haven was that of Sunday, 18th September, 1853. A large number of ships had taken shelter at Dale Roads from a westerly gale. During the night the wind changed to an easterly direction, leaving them on a lee shore. Many lost or dragged their anchors; some were intentionally run on the beach, others were driven against the rocks and more seriously damaged. Altogether, fourteen ships came ashore near Dale that night.

On 20th October, 1896, Tenby was struck by a particularly violent storm which demolished a considerable section of the pier and caused havoc among the shipping - mostly Brixham fishing smacks - sheltering in the harbour. Among the vessels dashed against the harbour wall was the cutter *Wasp* of Tenby, which had spent the earlier part of the year trawling in Carmarthen Bay. So severe was the damage sustained that she became a total loss.

Fortunately, most of the accidents which took place in harbour were relatively minor, involving, as in the case of the *Ant*, only loss of property. But no sailor could ever feel totally secure until he had actually set foot on dry land.

VIII; Death of a Veteran

"Lost off St. David's Head 25th April 1873." The simple statement in the Port of Milford Register records the end of the career of the sailing vessel *Anne & Mary*. The entry states that she had been registered there on 1st June, 1849, as a single masted and single decked sloop of 15 tons. Her dimensions were: length 35.5ft., breadth 10.7ft., and depth of hold 5.5ft.. She was carvel built, with a square stern and running bowsprit, but no figurehead. In 1849 she was jointly owned by John Williams of Solva, merchant, and David Williams of Drim (Goodwick), farmer, each of whom held 32 shares in the vessel.

A very ordinary and insignificant craft! Except in one respect; *Anne & Mary* had been built at Newport in the year 1762. For one hundred and eleven years she had ploughed her way around the treacherous waters of West Wales and the Bristol Channel. She would have been a frequent visitor to most of the harbours and isolated beaches of North Pembrokeshire - in her time she would have known several of them as her home port - and she would have been equally familiar with the creeks and quays of Milford Haven.

Even older was the ketch *Abbey* of Bristol; built in 1744, she was wrecked on the Goscar rock in January 1861 while on a voyage from Bridgwater to Haverfordwest with a cargo of timber and bricks. The *Pembrokeshire Herald* of 9th January considered that it was fortunate that the career of this ancient - and, it was suggested, unseaworthy - vessel had ended without loss of life. Her master Captain Bull and crew were rescued by the Tenby lifeboat.

By contrast the New Quay sloop *Friends* was barely a year old at the time of her loss. In late September, 1825, she was homeward bound from Milford with a cargo of culm. Approaching Ramsey Sound, when off Porth Llisky, she sprang a leak. The *Carmarthen Journal* of 30th September recounts how the master and boy who formed her crew each took hold of an oar and, using it as a support, made for the shore. The strength of the tides proved too much for the master who was drowned; but the boy, after stripping off most of his clothes, managed to struggle ashore. The ill-fated *Friends*, at 8 tons register and thirty feet in length, was one of the smallest of the coastal traders as well as one of the least fortunate.

Of the first quarter century of the existence of *Anne & Mary* no official records remain; however, in accordance with the Shipping Registration Act of 1786, she was registered for the first time at the Port of Cardigan on 1st February, 1787, as a sloop of 17 tons. She is mentioned as belonging to Abercastle in a letter, dated 18th December, 1800, from Peter Williams, a Bristol merchant, to his nephew John Williams who was then farming Trearched in Llanrhian parish. Further correspondence between the two men suggests there was fairly regular sea communication between Abercastle and Bristol (sometimes in Fishguard ships) and that wheat, barley, oats and butter were being exported from Abercastle at that time. Other topics mentioned include the price of corn and butter, and the advantages of shipping corn in sacks as opposed to loose in the hold.

Anne & Mary was probably at that time owned by the Morgan family of Abercastle. During the 1770s, William Morgan, mariner, had taken on a number of apprentices for training in seamanship and navigation. By 1790 he had been succeeded by John Morgan, merchant and mariner, presumably his son, who had carried on the practice well into the nineteenth century.

Anne & Mary was again registered at Cardigan on 29th June, 1825. By then she was owned by Martha Morgan, spinster, of Abercastle. Miss Morgan owned shares in a number of other vessels (a common practice) including eight in the 144 ton *Valiant* and four in the 130 ton *Venerable*, both brigs of Newport. She also held six shares in the 51 ton sloop *Princess Royal* and four in the 156 ton brigantine *Thomas*, both of Fishguard.

In 1825 James Rowland was master of the *Anne & Mary*. It was not until 26th September, 1840, that he was replaced at Milford by Thomas Davies. Presumably, throughout the early years of the century, much of her time was spent carrying culm and limestone to Abercastle. Records reveal that during 1845 the sloop had loaded two cargoes, each of 22 tons of culm, at Nolton. Thomas Davies, of Abercastle, appears to have been the merchant as well as the master on these occasions.

Martha Morgan died in 1834, aged 66. William Morgan of Trefin, the executor of her estate, continued to operate the vessel for several years. *Anne & Mary* was eventually sold to John Williams of Solva and David Williams of Drim, but it was a further two years before the change of ownership was registered at the Custom House, Milford.

John Williams of Tanyrallt was by far the most important corn and culm merchant in Solva at this time; some time earlier he had taken over a large culm and limeburning business from Michael James. To service this trade he purchased a number of small coasting vessels which feature regularly in the Folkeston Colliery records. *Anne & Mary*, with Thomas John as master, was among them - she also made at least one voyage to Goodwick with culm for David Williams.

The voyages to Nolton would have represented only a small fraction of those made each year. Most of the journeys which *Anne & Mary* undertook would have been to what is sometimes referred to as 'Milford River' - the upper reaches of Milford Haven - for culm and limestone. And there would perhaps have been a few voyages to Saundersfoot for culm and along the coast to South Wales to fetch coal more suited to household use.

The 1840s had been a time of prosperity in corn production in Pembrokeshire, a prosperity in which the limeburning industry shared. But the 1850s saw a sudden reduction in the amount of lime required. Agriculture was in decline, and other, newer fertilizers were becoming available. John Williams no longer needed so many ships, and on 27th March, 1863, he disposed of his shares in *Anne & Mary* to David Williams.

According to *Slater's Directory* of 1856, David Williams of Goodwick was a coal merchant; he was also one of the two lime burners listed for Fishguard and Goodwick. Under her new owner, *Anne & Mary* continued to carry culm and limestone from Milford; by the 1860s other cargoes were becoming difficult to obtain. During the second half of 1867, the vessel made seven voyages from Milford to Fishguard with culm and limestone; her crew by now consisted of only two men - Richard James aged 70 and David James aged 40, both of Dinas.

There was obviously little profit to be made. With the advent of steamships like the *Prince Cadwgan* of Aberaeron, which established in 1864 a fortnightly service with Bristol via Fishguard and Solva, one source of income was cut off. There was little demand for lime and that affected the culm trade. When an offer to purchase *Anne & Mary* was made in 1870, David Williams was probably delighted to accept.

The purchaser and final owner of the sloop was William Watts. He lived at Abereiddi, which was a centre for the one trade for which the future seemed bright - the slate trade. Slate quarrying on a major scale had begun at Abereiddi by 1840. For a time it had prospered, the slate being exported in small craft from the beach. But Abereiddi was an open bay, exposed to the west and with dangerous offshore reefs. It could never be developed as a proper harbour.

A mile or so to the north was the relatively sheltered inlet of Porthgain; as yet undeveloped it was used only by the occasional sloop with a cargo of culm or limestone for the neighbouring farms. Here, in 1851, a rudimentary harbour was constructed, protected by two short stone piers. A tramway was laid to carry slate from Abereiddi to the new wharf at Porthgain, and a second slate quarry was opened a short distance to the west of the harbour.

Periods of prosperity alternated with spells of depression. During the 1860s the quarries were taken over by the *St. Bride's Slate and Slab Company*. Once again success seemed assured: slates were being exported far afield, and no doubt William Watts saw the chance of profit.

The hoped-for boom did not materialise - at least not then. It was to be over a quarter of a century before it arrived under a company known as *United Stone Firms*. Even then it was based on a brickworks and particularly on granite quarries, both of which were opened at Porthgain in 1889, rather than on the black slates of Abereiddi. It was not until the early twentieth century that the modern harbour was built, providing a brief final flourish for the sloops before steam took over. But, by then, William Watts and *Anne & Mary* were both long gone.

During the second half of 1870, under her new owner, *Anne & Mary* made just seven voyages from Milford to Fishguard with limestone and culm. By 1873 conditions had still not improved; the crew now consisted of only James Jenkins and fifteen years old Thomas Jenkins, probably his son.

On 1st April, 1873, *Anne & Mary* began what was to be her last season; between that date and 18th April she made four voyages from Milford to

Abercastle. A week later, on her fifth voyage, the little sloop foundered near St. David's Head.

The local papers make no mention of her loss; the records give no reason for her sinking. There is no evidence of bad weather, as far as is known she struck no rock. Perhaps she was just worn out after a century of toil. The precise details of her end may remain just one of the minor mysteries of the sea.

A sad end for a grand old lady; veteran of perhaps three thousand voyages. But it was a nobler fate than to end her days a rotting skeleton on a mud-flat in a creek in Milford Haven; a fate that befell many of her sisters in the late nineteenth century. The sea also claimed her owner, William Watts, who was drowned at Swansea some four years later.

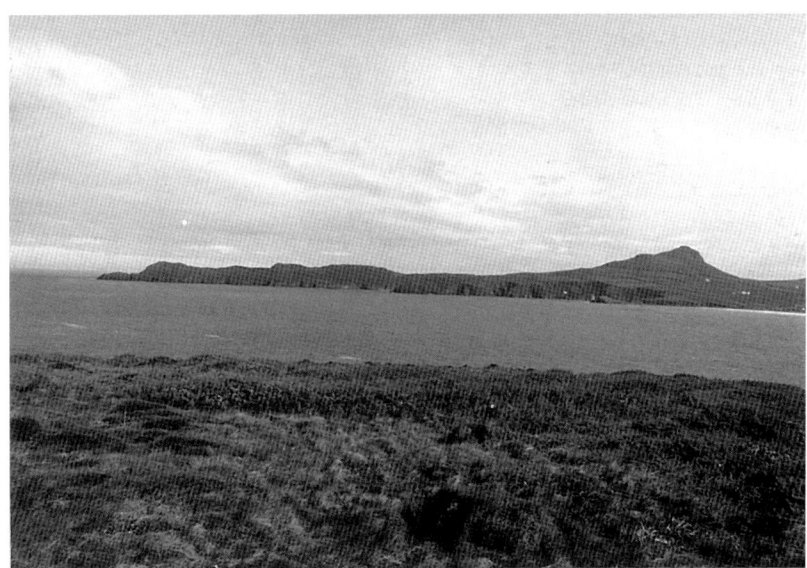

12. St. David's Head and Carnllidi from the south side of Whitesands Bay.

List of Shipwrecks

The list comprises sloops and similar craft, registered in West Wales, which were lost around the Pembrokeshire coast.

Name of Ship	Home Port	Register	Rig	Ton	Built	Year	Details of loss	Date of loss	p.
ABEONA	Cardigan	C52/07	sm	30	St D'maels	1852	lost Anglas Point Fishguard Bay	26.10.1859	21
ACTIVE	Cardigan	C37/12	sl	26	Cardigan	1826	lost all hands in Ramsey Sound	31.10.1846	
ACTIVE	St Dogmaels	C52/01	sm	29	Milford	1838	lost on St Anns Head	13.5.1860	
AID	Cardigan	C36/91	sl	25	Cardigan	1829	lost off Ramsey Island	13.9.1869	
ALERT	Newport	C37/05	sl	23	Newport	1835	lost St Davids Head	3.4.1861	
ALICE	St Davids	M40/12	sm	29	Milford	1840	stranded at Little Haven	22.3.1878	
ALLIGATOR	Solva	M37/32	sm	21	Lawrenny	1837	wrecked Penpleidiau St Brides Bay	14.9.1858	13
ANN	Cardigan	C45/02	sl	24	New Quay	1821	foundered Fishguard Bay	18.6.1884	
ANN	Hakin	M29/09	sl	32	Milford	1829	lost off Strumble Head all perished	1835	
ANN	Manorbier	M29/12	sl	24	Lawrenny	1814	lost Tenby Bay	26.9.1833	
ANN	St Dogmaels	C37/21	sl	31	Cardigan	1818	total wreck near Jack Sound	17.7.1849	26
ANN & MARY	Dinas	C55/11	sm	30	New Quay	1847	stranded total wreck Pwllgwaelod	16.9.1880	
ANN DAVIES	New Quay	A63/12	sm	21	Traethgwyn	1863	wrecked in Jack Sound	9.8.1880	17
ANN ELIZA	Llansantffraid	A62/15	sm	44	L'santffraid	1862	wrecked 'Ramsey Sound nr Milford'	11.5.1877	
ANN JONES	St Dogmaels	C53/03	sm	27	St D'maels	1853	run down 4 miles off South Bishop	Feb 1856	28
ANNA MARIA	Carmarthen	L50/01	sl	28	St Clears	1834	lost near Pendine	1.10.1863	
ANNE	Fishguard	C36/40	sl	22	Fishguard	1830	lost Strumble with all hands	Mar 1858	
ANNE & BETSEY	Cardigan	C26/64	sl	44	New Quay	1826	wrecked Jack Sound	21.9.1838	
ANNE & MARY	Abercastle	M49/07	sl	15	Newport	1762	lost off St Davids Head	25.4.1873	42
ANNIE	Tenby	M90/02	k	23	Dartmouth	1890	sank Tenby	27.3.1916	
ANT	Pembroke Dock	M55/06	sl	24	Mevagissey	1830	lost all hands Sprinkle - St Davids	Mar 1865	12
ANTELOPE	St Ishmaels	M47/05	sm	20	Milford	1827	wrecked Sandy Haven	1.2.1876	38
ATLANTIC	Milford	M51/11	c	22	Scilly Isles	1837	foundered at Goultrop	25.11.1875	31
AURORA	New Quay	C36/63	sl	48	New Quay	1835	gone to pieces in Ramsey Sound	3.7.1847	
BETSEY	Borth	A27/13	sl	40	C'then	1799	totally lost on North Bishops	29.6.1846	9
BETSEY	Pembroke	M36/32	sm	78	Pembroke	1828	lost on voyage from Wexford	5.5.1829	39
								Mar 1838	

46

Name of Ship	Home Port	Register	Rig	Ton	Built	Year	Details of loss	Date of loss	p.
BETSEY	St Davids	M19/01	sl	28	Milford	1819	lost near Porthclais	c 1830	9
BREESE	Tenby	M50/10	sm	28	Cork	1839	run down off Caldey I	18.8.1866	
BRISTOL TRADER	Fishguard	A53/21	sl	28	Derwenlas	1790	wrecked & broken up at Fishguard	1864	21
BRITANNIA	Dinas	M68/02	sm	30	Cardigan	1797	lost off St Davids Head	19.8.1881	40
BRITON	Cardigan	C45/10	sl	37	New Quay	1839	lost off Strumble Head	10.9.1859	
BROTHERS	Borth	A52/06	sm	35	Morfa ucha	1828	foundered 9 miles off Strumble Hd	1.6.1864	
BROTHERS	Pembroke Ferry	M39/22	sm	35	Pem Ferry	1839	wrecked Tenby	1.11.1859	
CANDACE	Aberystwyth	A50/13	k	34	A'ystwyth	1850	foundered collision St Govans Hd	Dec 1892	
CATHERINE	St Davids	A64/24	sm	16	Ynyslas	1864	destroyed by fire Porthclais Harbour	4.1.1876	41
CHRISTINE	Milford	M03/01	k	68	Pem Dock	1903	wr passage Wexford to Milford	16.2.1906	
COMET	Aberystwyth	A53/16	sl	33	Cardigan	1816	wrecked Aberfelin crew saved	6.8.1860	12
COMMERCE	New Quay	C36/71	sl	18	New Quay	1830	lost in Ramsey Sound	6.8.1844	8
COMMERCE	St Dogmaels	C51/03	sm	32	New Quay	1844	totally wrecked Goodwick Sands	10.11.1872	
CONNIVUM	Dinas	C57/04	sl	23	Conway	1840	wrecked at Pwllgwaelod	2.11.1873	
CORNWALLIS	Tenby	M30/08	sl	46	Bristol	1805	lost Saundersfoot Bay	21.5.1832	
COUNTESS OF LISBURN	Aberystwyth	A54/04	sm	30	A'ystwyth	1836	foundered with all hands on voyage Milford – Aberystwyth	c 1865	
COURIER	St Davids	M59/02	sm	21	Hakin	1859	wrecked Porthclais	18.10.1879	34
CURLEW	Fishguard	M48/07	sm	28	Milford	1848	foundered off Pembrokeshire coast	21.7.1868	37
CYMRO	Moylegrove	C93/01	sl	32	Milford	1888	lost in Milford River	14.11.1902	
DART	Aberystwyth	A57/30	sl	47	Bridgwater	1845	stranded near Strumble Head	17.3.1863	
DAVID	St Dogmaels	C37/31	sl	26	Newport	1830	sank at anchor nr Grassholm Ramsey Sound	16.12.1882	
DILIGENCE	Aberdyfi	A25/15	sl	29	Derwenlas	1809	abandoned nr Grassholm crew saved	4.1.1843	15
DILIGENCE	Borth	A53/17	sm	36	Newcastle	1835	wrecked Musselwick St Brides Bay	20.4.1868	
DISPATCH	Llansantffraid	A29/09	sl	42	L'santffraid	1805	totally lost in St Brides Bay	4.7.1829	
DOLPHIN	Aberporth	M36/42	sl	45	Milford	1828	lost 4m NW Cardigan Head	22.7.1878	
DOLPHIN	Cardigan	C31/05	sm	28	New Quay	1804	lost in Ramsey Sound	31.7.1831	
DOVE	Moylegrove	C29/05	sl	15	Cardigan	1819	lost at Goultrop Road	8.10.1835	
EAGLE	Borth	A41/06	sl	23	A'ystwyth	1786	wrecked Freshwater West	8.11.1841	
ELEANOR GRACE	Llangrannog	A53/09	sl	23	Celbach	1838	foundered near Strumble Head	5.8.1884	
ELIZA	Llanelli	L42/07	sm	27	L'shipping	1834	wrecked Bluckspool near Linney Hd	21.11.1863	37
	Haverfordwest	M36/27	sm	39	Lawrenny	1819	wrecked by collision Milford	31.10.1859	41

47

Name of Ship	Home Port	Register	Rig	Ton	Built	Year	Details of loss	Date	p.
ELIZABETH	Newport	C40/07	sl	28	Newport	1839	sank in Jack Sound	18.4.1867	
ELIZABETH & MARY	Newport	C25/102	sl	60	Newport	1792	lost near Milford	11.2.1828	
ELIZABETH & MARY	Newport	C56/02	sm	20	Pem Dock	1854	lost on Strumble Head	19.2.1861	10
ELIZABETH MARIA	Aberaeron	A48/14	sl	33	Llangrannog	1827	lost St Brides Bay	1848	
ELLEN	Aberaeron	A52/18	sm	26	Aberaeron	1852	totally wrecked St Brides Bay	11.9.1866	
ELLEN	Milford	M82/02	sm	27	Liverpool	1808	stranded Cardigan Bay total wreck	26.9.1884	
ELLEN	St Dogmaels	C59/04	sl	40	Ulverston	1842	wrecked (lost) in Ramsey Sound	28.8.1860	
ELLEN GWENLLIAN	Haverfordwest	M58/09	sm	26	Saunders-foot	1847	lost near Milford	22.8.1868	37
EXLEY	Newport	C61/06	sl	30	Hull	1840	lost on rocks at Pencaer Strumble	3.4.1871	12
FAME	Aberystwyth	A27/05	sl	39	A'ystwyth	1789	run down off St Anns Light 3am	14.8.1828	15
FANNY & BETSEY	Pembroke	M30/10	sm	36	Land-shipping	1830	lost with crew on voyage from Wicklow to Pembroke	Jan 1832	
FANNY ANNE	Newport	C25/93	sl	23	Newport	1801	lost off Milford	22.5.1841	
FAWN	Fishguard	C96/02	sm	34	Pem Dock	1873	lost in Jack Sound	25.4.1903	
FIDELITY	Fishguard	C26/07	sl	24	Fishguard	1807	lost near St Anns Light	21.7.1846	36
FLORA	Newport	C25/118	sl	29	Newport	1795	lost off Milford	1829	
FLOWER OF OVERGANG	Fishguard	M58/04	sm	24	Brixham	1828	total wreck Carreg Onnen near Strumble crew saved in boat	20.9.1869	
FLY	Newport	C63/03	sm	24	unknown	–	sank off Strumble Head crew lost	24.4.1873	
FRANCES	Newport	C37/69	sl	22	Aberporth	1808	wrecked Middle Sledge off Abereiddi	28.5.1863	
FRIENDS	Llansantffraid	A48/13	sm	39	Aberaeron	1838	broken on rocks St Davids Hd	24.10.1865	
FRIENDS	New Quay	C25/52	sl	8	New Quay	1824	lost with master Porthllisky	Sep 1825	42
FRIENDS	New Quay	C36/54	sl	25	New Quay	1835	lost at Strumble Head	3.6.1851	
FRIENDS	St Dogmaels	M56/01	sl	28	Foreign	–	lost off Caldey I	Oct 1867	
GEORGE	Pembroke Dock	M45/10	sl	41	Fife	1793	lost near St Govans Head	1846	
GEORGE THE FOURTH	Carmarthen	L36/21	sm	36	Hereford	1825	lost off Tenby	2.7.1838	
GIPSY	Pembroke Dock	M46/14	sm	36	Lawrenny	1837	lost off St Davids Head	25.9.1862	
GOOD HOPE	Cardigan	C37/33	sl	22	New Quay	1828	lost St Anns Head master drowned	23.11.1858	

48

Name of Ship	Home Port	Register	Rig	Ton	Built	Year	Details of loss	Date	p.
GOOD HOPE	New Quay	C40/05	sl	27	A'ystwyth	1825	struck rock sank Ramsey Sound	26.10.1867	
GWENDOLINE	Milford	M87/01	k	33	Milford	1887	lost by collision St Brides Bay	16.9.1891	
HANDY	Milford	M65/01	dy	26	unknown		sank in Haven	1867	8
HANNAH	Milford	M65/04	sl	13	Aberaeron	1829	lost near Solva	12.8.1870	
HARRIET & ANN	Llanelli	L48/04	sl	30	C'then	1825	lost 6 miles off Milford	25.7.1849	
HERO	Carmarthen	L29/05	sl	51	C'then	1803	wr nr Pendine – master's wife lost	Nov 1830	
HOPE	Aberystwyth	A25/32	sl	56	Craiglas	1821	lost near Tenby	25.4.1833	
HOPE	Cardigan	C37/18	sl	17	New Quay	1803	totally wrecked Strumble Head	8.10.1865	
HOPE	Fishguard	C25/45	sl	35	L A'colwin	1805	foundered off Bishops & Clerks	3.9.1826	
HOPE	Newport	C25/122	sl	21	Newport	1808	lost all hands Goultrop	Mar 1827	
HOPEWELL	Aberystwyth	C26/01	sl	61	Derwenlas	1826	foundered off St Govans crew lost	26.12.1833	
HOPEWELL	Cardigan	C47/05	sl	35	L'grannog	1810	lost Horse Rock Ramsey Sound	30.9.1870	
HOPEWELL	Newport	C42/07	sl	18	New Quay	1828	lost at Fishguard	14.8.1852	
INDUSTRIOUS	Solva	M38/18	sm	17	Milford	1799	lost in Jack Sound crew lost	11.5.1839	17
INDUSTRY *	Aberystwyth	A35/23	sl	63	A'ystwyth	1846	sank Musselwick Milford Haven	25.11.1838	40
INDUSTRY	Pembroke Dock	M58/05	sm	18	Caernarfon	1843	lost off St Anns Head	3.2.1861	
JANE	Newport	M43/08	sm	18	Tenby	1809	lost at Jack Sound	Nov 1873	
JANE	Solva	M33/05	sl	28	Solva	1837	lost Jack Sound	16.10.1837	17
JANE & CATHERINE	Newport	C64/03	sl	29	Conway		lost in Ramsey Sound	12.9.1869	
JANE & MARGARET	Newport	C79/02	sl	25	L'santffraid (Denbigh)	1859	totally wrecked at Newport	16.8.1879	
JANE ELLEN	Aberystwyth	A51/11	sm	35	A'ystwyth	1851	foundered off St Davids Head	29.1.1874	26
JENNY	St Dogmaels	C33/09	sl	23	New Quay	1792	lost at Newport	22.10.1840	
JOHN	Fishguard	C53/02	sl	17	Milford	1828	lost in Fishguard Bay	26.5.1867	
JOHN & GRACE	Fishguard	M69/10	sl	29	Dartmouth	1802	wrecked on Goodwick Sands	10.11.1872	8
JOHN & MARY	Dinas	M55/05	sl	18	Llanelli	1828	lost Ramsey Sound	Aug 1868	
JOHN JAMES	New Quay	A70/12	sl	30	Flint	1859	wrecked foundered Jack Sound	13.2.1901	
KING	Haverfordwest	M33/24	sl	22	Pem Dock	1831	lost in Jack Sound	1836	16
LIBERTY	Haverfordwest	M30/26	sl	69	Hook	1810	totally lost Crow Rock	30.4.1831	12
LILLY	Fishguard	C52/05	sm	34	Bideford	1798	lost off Strumble Head	12.9.1868	
LION *	St Dogmaels	C37/50	sl	28	Cardigan	1810	stranded at Fishguard	10.10.1862	
LIVELY	Borth	A48/07	sl	28	L Aberarth	1826	sprang leak foundered Newport Bar	17.12.1849	

49

Name of Ship	Home Port	Register	Rig	Ton	Built	Year	Details of loss	Date	p.
LIZZIE	Tenby	M36/04	sm	49	Milford	1836	came on shore Freshwater West	15.3.1839	
LIZZIE ANNIE	Fishguard	M67/06	c	25	Milford	1867	lost at Ramsey Sound	22.8.1891	
MAJOR NANNEY	New Quay	A56/18	sl	43	Pwllheli	1841	stranded total wreck St Govans Hd	1.4.1878	
MARGARET	St Davids	M54/17	sl	17	Lawrenny	1849	lost near St Brides Stack	25.7.1893	
MARGARET & ANN	Tresaith	C77/03	sl	33	Cardigan	1877	lost Friday night by St Anns Head	14.3.1919	
MARGARET & JANE	Llanddewi Aberarth	C41/16	sm	30	Aberllong	1841	foundered in St Georges Channel crew perished	20.11.1846	
MARGARET LLOYD	Aberystwyth	A54/08	dy	53	A'ystwyth	1854	lost off Cardigan with all 4 hands	26.10.1859	21
MARGARET MARY	Borth	A46/15	sm	31	A'ystwyth	1842	lost deep water Fishguard Bay	20.12.1853	
MARGARETTA	Aberaeron	C68/01	sm	25	Lawrenny	1842	stranded on rocks Pwllgwaelod	11.5.1897	
MARIETTA	Aberystwyth	A48/35	sl	56	New Quay	1831	run down 40 miles NE South Bishop	10.5.1850	
MARTHA	Lawrenny	M43/09	sm	31	Lawrenny	1843	wrecked off Saundersfoot	Jan 1867	
MARTHA JANE	St Davids	M72/02	c	17	Cosheston	1872	wrecked on Bitches Ramsey Sound	19.3.1894	17
MARY	Aberporth	C26/54	sl	24	Cardigan	1791	lost at Fishguard	10.9.1827	
MARY	Aberporth	C37/67	sl	23	Cardigan	1837	sunk collision nr St Anns crew lost	23.7.1854	27
MARY	Aberystwyth	A43/04	sl	60	A'ystwyth	1805	ashore Broad Haven went to pieces	16.7.1853	
MARY	Newport	C25/41	sl	53	Newport	1819	chain parted drifted ashore Tenby	Nov 1834	
MARY	Pembroke Dock	M53/07	sl	45	Lawrenny	1802	lost in Jack Sound	19.12.1853	18
MARY	St Dogmaels	C37/74	sl	18	Brynhenlle	1833	wrecked at Abercastle	24.12.1895	
MARY	St Dogmaels	C50/07	sm	27	Lancaster	1842	lost collision off Strumble Head	5.4.1859	25
MARY ANN	Aberystwyth	A52/10	sl	50	Towyn	1817	lost at St Govans Head	3.11.1857	
MARY ANN	Borth	A40/03	sl	52	Garreg	1812	wrecked Freshwater West	20.7.1841	
MARY ANN	Hakin	M33/23	sm	29	Milford	1829	lost in Dale Roads	Feb 1838	
MARY ANN	Milford	M66/04	sm	25	Milford	1866	wrecked Abermawr	14.5.1906	
MARY ELLEN	Aberystwyth	A48/23	sm	35	A'ystwyth	1848	struck Crow Rock sank deep water	4.8.1849	
MOLLY	Aberporth	C37/23	sl	22	Cardigan	1802	lost at St Davids Sound	12.6.1841	
MOLLY LLOYD	St Dogmaels	C25/136	sl	21	L'santffraid	1799	lost Ramsey Sound	15.9.1842	26
MORNING STAR	Aberystwyth	A36/13	sm	47	A'ystwyth	1827	wrecked Cardigan Bar, crew lost	26.10.1859	21
MORNING STAR	St Dogmaels	C26/39	sl	16	Aberaeron	1800	lost Blackpool near Milford Harbour	May 1837	26
MYRA	Fishguard	A37/47	sm	22	New Quay	1832	lost in Jack Sound	3.1.1868	

Name of Ship	Home Port	Register	Rig	Ton	Built	Year	Details of loss	Date	p.
NEW DOLPHIN	Llansantffraid	A29/03	sl	20	L'santffraid	1829	lost off Strumble Head	12.3.1848	
NEW HOPE	Aberystwyth	A53/29	sl	32	New Quay	1828	sprung leak, foundered off Milford	5.10.1861	
NEW HOPE	Fishguard	C37/28	sl	16	Tresaith	1827	lost in Ramsey Sound	9.10.1845	
NEW MILFORD	Cosheston	M65/03	sm	24	Cosheston	1863	wrecked Shoe Ramsey Sound	10.12.1868	8
OAK	Newport	C59/01	f	33	Queensferry	1840	lost (holed and beached Newport)	Jun 1860	
OCEAN	Llangrannog	C36/66	sl	33	Aberaeron	1827	total wreck on Cardigan Bar	2.10.1895	
OCEAN	New Quay	C44/03	sl	28	Celbach	1844	foundered near Caldey I	29.10.1865	
OSPRAY	Aberystwyth	A47/05	sm	33	Aberaeron	1836	foundered off Milford crew saved	12.9.1871	
OSPREY	New Quay	C36/89	sl	47	New Quay	1835	lost Ramsey Island	10.6.1865	
PEARL	Pembroke	M53/10	sm	28	Lawrenny	1853	wrecked St Catherines I Tenby	3.8.1880	35
PEGGY	St Dogmaels	C26/31	sl	27	Cardigan	1782	wrecked Cardigan Bar	30.9.1841	25
PEGGY	St Dogmaels	C48/02	sl	19	St D'maels	1804	totally wrecked Cardigan Bar	20.10.1873	
PENELOPE	Fishguard	L50/05	sm	27	St Clears	1837	foundered at sea off Stackpole	28.3.1879	
PENRHYN CASTLE	Aberporth	C42/01	sm	44	Lawrenny	1839	run down by mail steamer near St Anns Head	30.9.1873	28
PERFECT	Milford	M04/05	c	20	B'lingsea	1866	totally wrecked Fishguard	31.7.1909	
PILGRIM	Solva	M40/11	sl	18	Milford	1808	lost with crew St Brides Bay	28.9.1845	8
PRICE JONES	Newport	C61/08	f	24	Flint	1859	foundered in Ramsey Sound	12.9.1884	
PRINCESS LOUISE *	Little Haven	M90/05	sm	25	Sitting- bourne	1871	wrecked near Dale (restored as ketch)	6.11.1890	
PROGRESS	Aberystwyth	A63/01	k	80	A'ystwyth	1863	foundered Fishguard Bay	26.3.1898	
PROVIDENCE	Cardigan	C34/13	sl	24	St D'maels	1776	lost at Goodwick	7.9.1838	
PROVIDENCE	St Dogmaels	C26/33	sl	29	Newport	1777	lost 'Jack Sound near St Davids'	9.7.1848	
PUNCH	Newport	M69/04	sm	24	Milford	1851	lost 20 miles NNE Strumble Head	6.12.1877	26
QUEEN OF TRUMPS	Fishguard	C55/05	sl	33	Pwllheli	1836	wrecked near Fishguard	1861	
RACHEL	Cardigan	C36/16	sl	25	Celbach	1836	foundered off Cardigan	6.10.1873	
RACHEL	Cardigan	C36/35	sl	33	Cardigan	1836	lost off Cardigan with crew	28.10.1843	
RANGER	Tenby	M50/08	c	20	Scilly Is	1823	lost at Tenby	1853	
RAPID	Aberporth	C40/11	sl	25	Cardigan	1840	foundered at Fishguard Roads	28.2.1884	
RECHABITE	Fishguard	M40/08	sm	19	Lawrenny	1840	sank Ramsey Sound	4.9.1861	29
RESOLUTION	Llansantffraid	A25/19	sl	41	A'ystwyth	1805	run down off Strumble Hd	9.10.1833	
RETRIEVER	St Dogmaels	C55/01	sl	44	Liverpool	1850	wrecked Old Castle Head Tenby	15.10.1869	26

51

Name of Ship	Home Port	Register	Rig	Ton	Built	Year	Details of loss	Date	p.
RICHARD & MARY	Newport	C49/06	sm	18	Pembroke Dock	1848	wrecked Betws Point Fishguard	13.10.1854	12
ROBUST	Borth	A42/12	sl	25	L Aberarth	1797	wrecked East Island, Abercastle	18.10.1854	
ROYAL OAK	Aberporth	C37/19	sl	23	New Quay	1811	wrecked Newport	May 1865	34
ROYAL OAK	New Quay	C24/08	sl	10	New Quay	1814	lost near Milford	1831	
RUBY	Aberystwyth	A56/05	dy	38	Dumbarton	1828	lost near Strumble Head	12.2.1859	
RUBY	Cardigan	C49/05	sl	22	Cardigan	1839	wrecked near S Bishop crew lost	9.6.1851	25
SAINT DAVID	St Davids	M26/10	sl	25	Neyland	1826	lost Caerbwdi	1828	
SARAH ANN	Cardigan	M81/12	sm	24	Castle Pill	1881	wrecked near Porthgain total loss	12.9.1909	
SEAFLOWER	Fishguard	C25/46	sl	21	Fishguard	1789	lost off Strumble Head	31.7.1839	
SEVEN BROTHERS	Tenby	M44/11	sm	29	Bideford	1834	totally lost Skomer I master lost	21.3.1846	
SISTERS	Porthgain	M29/16	sm	27	Cork	1811	driven on shore Ramsey Sound	27.8.1829	8
SOPHIA	Llangrannog	C39/15	sl	39	Greenock	1839	lost off Strumble Head	13.11.1860	
SUSSEX	Aberystwyth	A46/05	sm	42	Hastings	1835	lost on Cardigan Bar	6.11.1852	
SWANSEA TRADER	Borth	A59/32	sm	35	Bideford	1828	lost with crew off Dinas Head	26.10.1859	21
TAFF OF TWENTY TWO	Dinas	C45/01	sl	26	Cardiff	1822	lost at entrance to Cardigan river	29.10.1851	33
TAYLOR & NAYLOR	Newport	M68/07	sm	30	Wexford	1839	sunk total loss near Newport	Oct 1869	
TERESSA	St Ishmaels	M42/10	sm	22	Milford	1842	wrecked St Brides Bay	17.3.1851	
THOMAS	Aberaeron	A64/01	sm	26	Padstow	1859	lost collision off St Govans Head	Dec 1892	
THREE SISTERS	Aberaeron	C25/141	sl	33	New Quay	1813	wrecked near St Davids Head	5.7.1829	8
TIVY LASS	Cardigan	C40/26	sl	34	Cardigan	1840	wrecked near Musselwick Little Haven	6.8.1860	
TRUE BESS	St Davids	M56/10	sl	20	Aberaeron	1846	wrecked near Goultrop crew lost	25.10.1859	20
TRUE BRITON	St Dogmaels	C37/45	sl	16	Aberporth	1793	stranded Abercastle total loss	6.7.1856	
TURTLE DOVE	Milford	A48/08	sl	36	L Aberarth	1832	stranded Ramsey Sound.	6.5.1875	
TWO BROTHERS	St Davids	M58/20	sm	23	Merioneth	1834	lost off Ramsey	Mar 1872	
UNION	Cardigan	C52/04	sl	33	New Quay	1820	lost Cemaes Head	10.11.1866	26
UNION	St Davids	M81/04	sm	18	Lymington	1828	lost Caldey Roads	3.1.1866	
UNITY	Borth	A39/04	sl	17	Llangrannog	1813	foundered St Brides Bay crew saved	18.9.1852	
UNITY	Llangrannog	C39/09	sl	35	Ceibach	1839	totally wrecked Jack Sound	27.9.1876	

Name of Ship	Home Port	Register	Rig	Ton	Built	Year	Details of loss	Date	p.
VICTORIA	New Quay	C38/10	sl	38	Ceibach	1838	lost in Ramsey Sound	9.2.1845	8
VICTORY	Cardigan	C37/57	sl	51	Cardigan	1808	wrecked Cardigan Bar	Dec 1845	
WAFT	Tenby	M29/07	sl	24	L Aberarth	1813	lost St Govans	1836	14
WASP	New Quay	C39/16	sl	33	Ceibach	1839	lost Goultrop Road St Brides Bay	12.10.1870	
WASP	Tenby	M72/04	c	27	Falmouth	1848	wrecked Tenby Harbour total loss	20.10.1896	41
WATERLOO	Hakin	M34/06	sm	15	Milford	1816	lost on Skomer Island	19.6.1837	
WAVE QUEEN	Milford	M92/01	sm	34	L'hampton	1856	burned in Milford Haven	30.5.1893	41
WILLIAM	Pembroke	M28/05	sl	64	Pembroke	1828	wrecked near Fishguard crew saved	14.6.1833	
WILLIAM	St Davids	M61/03	sm	23	Pem Ferry	1861	lost off St Anns	3.8.1874	
WOMBWELL	Cardigan	C37/72	sl	20	Broadstairs	1818	missing voyage Cardigan – Milford	Jul 1839	12
WYRE MAID	Llanrhystyd	A48/18	sm	39	A'ystwyth	1848	lost all hands Milford Haven	18.10.1858	

Information on vessels based mainly on Shipping Registers;

A = Aberystwyth;   C = Cardigan;   L = Llanelli;   M = Milford

Register; The first two figures refer to the year of registration; the others give the entry number for that year. The entry M29/12 refers to entry number 12 for the Port of Milford in the year 1829. The number usually is that of the last registry of the ship. Milford Registers are complete from 1827, the others from 1824.

Home Port; In the early Cardigan Registers the subordinate port to which the ship belonged is sometimes stated. In most cases it represents the place where the majority of shares was owned. In almost all cases this information is taken from Shipping Registers and Transactions.

Rig;   c = cutter;   f = flat;   sl = sloop;   sm = smack   -   all single-masted, fore-and-aft rigged.
    dy = dandy;   k = ketch   -   both have short mizzen mast aft of mainmast.

Tonnage; The method of calculation changed several times, most importantly in 1836. As a rough guide the burthen (cargo capacity) until 1835 was equivalent to the registered tonnage; from 1836 the burthen was about 50% greater than the registered tonnage.

The list comprises sloops and similar craft registered in the West Wales ports which were lost off the Pembrokeshire coast. Information on date and location of wrecks is supplemented by other sources, including Crew Agreements and local newspapers.

Precise locations of wrecks are not normally recorded. Wreck locations on accompanying maps show only the general area in which a wreck took place. Ships whose names are shown in italics on maps are locally owned vessels mentioned in the text which have not been identified on the surviving Registers.

* Vessel wrecked or sunk (according to register) later salvaged and re-registered.

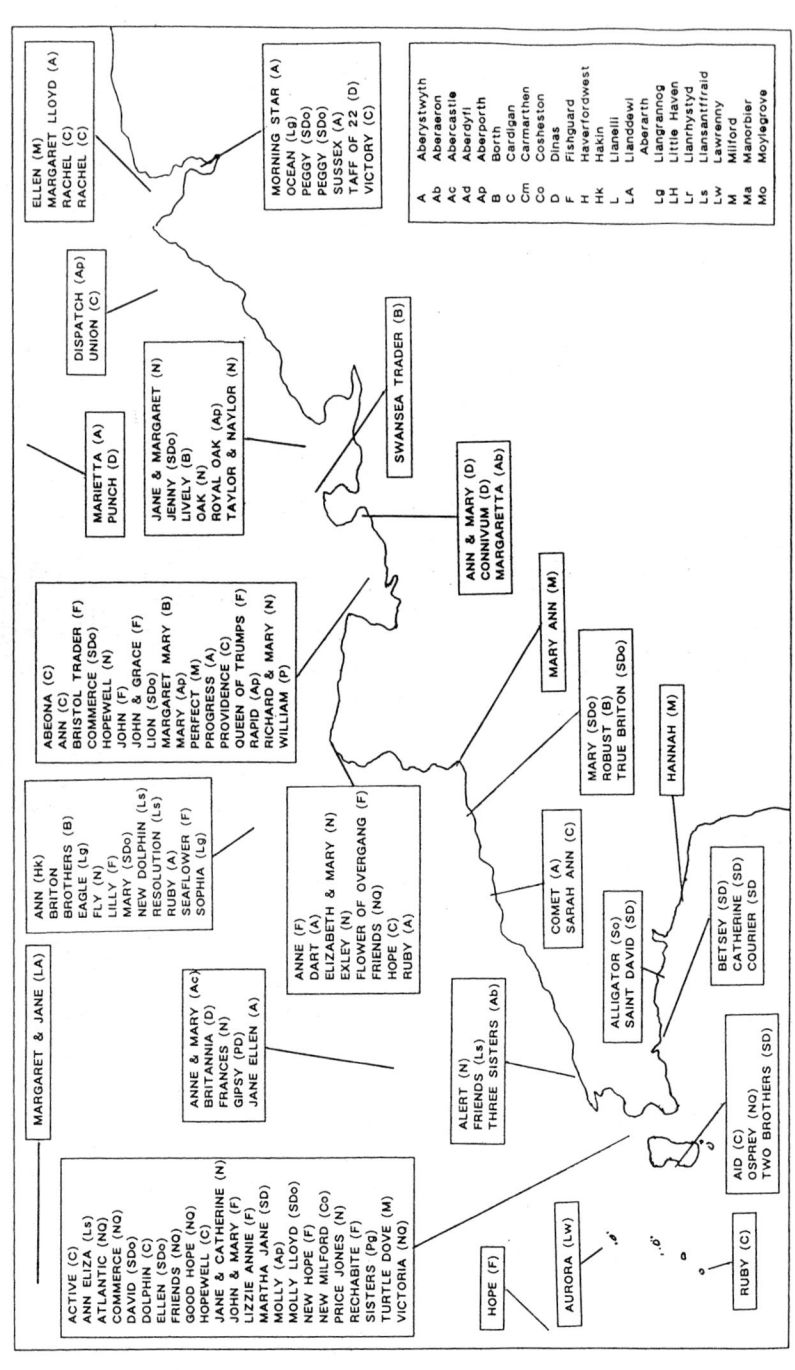

South Pembrokeshire Shipwrecks

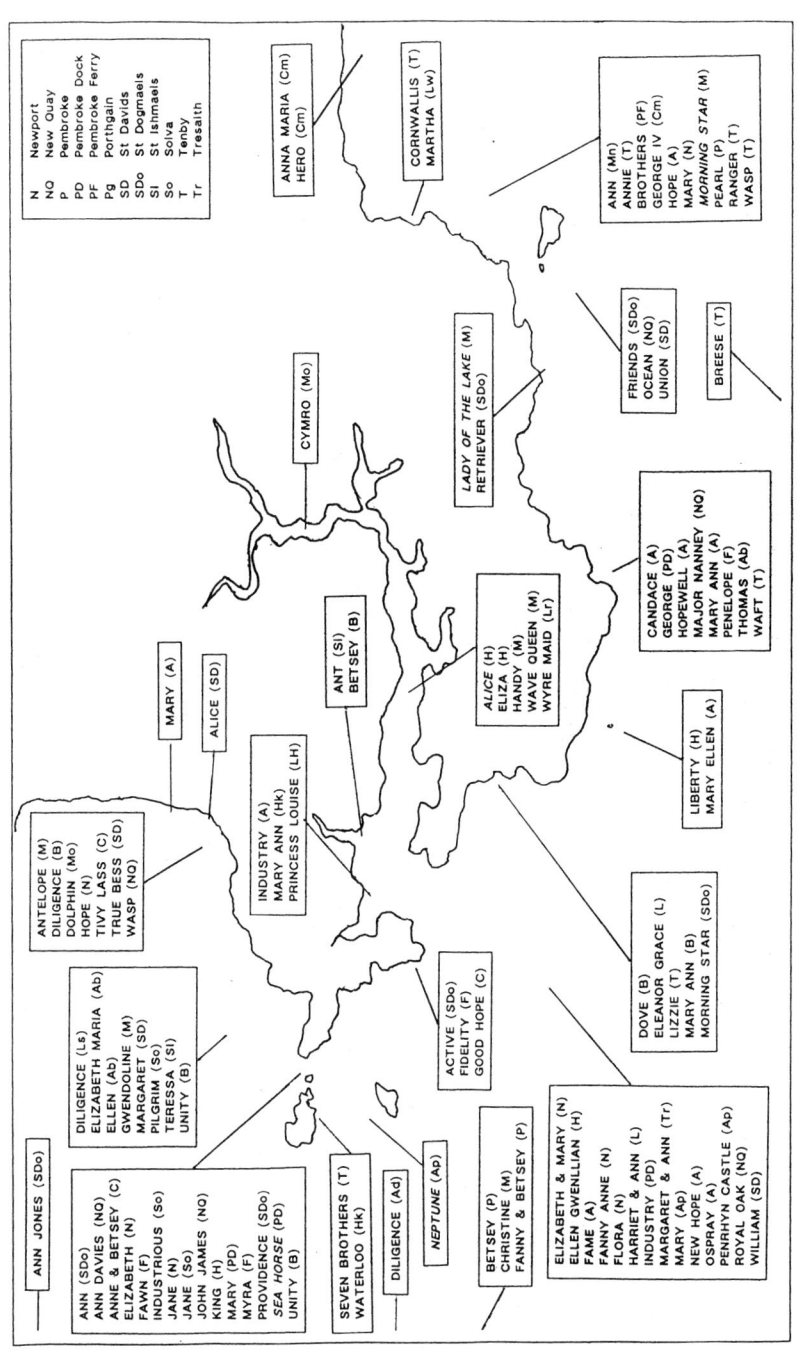

Bibliography

BENNETT, Tom: *Welsh Shipwrecks*, (I-III), (Haverfordwest, 1981-83).
BENNETT, Tom: *Fishguard Lifeboats: A Short History*, (Fishguard, 1984).
BENNETT, Tom: *Shipwrecks Around St David's*, (Newport, 1994).
BOWEN, E. G.: 'Seafaring along the Pembrokeshire Coast in the days of the Sailing Ships', *The Pembrokeshire Historian, No. 4*, (Haverfordwest, 1972).
GEORGE, Barbara: *Pembrokeshire Sea-Trading Before 1900*, (London, 1964).
GODDARD, Ted: *Pembrokeshire Shipwrecks*, (Swansea, 1984).
GREEN, Francis: 'Dewisland Coasters in 1751', *West Wales Historical Records*, VIII, (Carmarthen, 1919).
HAMPSON, Desmond G. & MIDDLETON, George W.: *The Story of the St. Davids Lifeboats*, (St. David's, 1974).
HARRIES, George: *Early Bristol Paddle-Steamer Shipwrecks*, (St. David's, 1993).
JAMES, David W.: *St. David's and Dewisland*, (Cardiff, 1981).
JENKINS, J. Geraint: *The Maritime Heritage of Dyfed*, (Cardiff, 1982).
JOHN, Brian: *Ports and Harbours of Pembrokeshire*, (Fishguard, 1974).
McKAY, K. D.: *A Vision of Greatness: The History of Milford 1790-1990*, (Haverfordwest, 1989).
MORRIS, Jeff: *Tenby Lifeboats*, (Tenby, 1987).
SCOTT, Richard S. L.: 'The Port of Fishguard', *Journal of the Pembrokeshire Historical Society*, No. 2, (Haverfordwest, 1988).

Newspapers:
Carmarthen Journal.
Pembrokeshire Herald & Advertiser.
Haverfordwest & Milford Haven Telegraph.
Dewsland & Kemes Guardian.